Psychological Treatment of
Patients With Chronic
Respiratory Disease

Clinical Health Psychology Series

Psychological Treatment of
Patients With Chronic
Respiratory Disease

SUSAN M. LABOTT

CLINICAL HEALTH PSYCHOLOGY SERIES

ELLEN A. DORNELAS, Series Editor

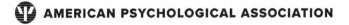 AMERICAN PSYCHOLOGICAL ASSOCIATION

The opinions and statements published are the responsibility of the authors, and such opinions and statements do not necessarily represent the policies of the American Psychological Association.

Published by
American Psychological Association
750 First Street, NE
Washington, DC 20002
https://www.apa.org

Order Department
https://www.apa.org/pubs/books
order@apa.org

In the U.K., Europe, Africa, and the Middle East, copies may be ordered from Eurospan
https://www.eurospanbookstore.com/apa
info@eurospangroup.com

Typeset in Charter and Interstate by Circle Graphics, Inc., Reisterstown, MD

Printer: Sheridan Books, Chelsea, MI
Cover Designer: Mercury Publishing Services, Inc., Rockville, MD

Library of Congress Cataloging-in-Publication Data

Names: Labott, Susan M., author.
Title: Psychological treatment of patients with chronic respiratory disease /
  Susan M. Labott.
Description: Washington, DC : American Psychological Association, [2020] |
  Series: Clinical health psychology | Includes bibliographical references and index.
Identifiers: LCCN 2020003202 (print) | LCCN 2020003203 (ebook) |
  ISBN 9781433832246 (paperback) | ISBN 9781433832253 (ebook)
Subjects: LCSH: Chronic diseases—Psychological aspects. | Neuropsychology. |
  Sick—Psychology.
Classification: LCC RC108 .L33 2020 (print) | LCC RC108 (ebook) |
  DDC 616/.044—dc23
LC record available at https://lccn.loc.gov/2020003202
LC ebook record available at https://lccn.loc.gov/2020003203

http://dx.doi.org/10.1037/0000189-000

Printed in the United States of America

10 9 8 7 6 5 4 3 2 1

To Jim

Contents

Series Foreword

Mental health practitioners working in medicine represent the vanguard of psychological practice. Scientific discovery and advances in medicine have been rapid in recent decades, and it has been a challenge for clinical health psychology practice to keep pace.

In a fast-changing field, and with a paucity of practice-based research, classroom models of health psychology practice often don't translate well to clinical care. All too often, health psychologists work in silos, with little appreciation of how advancement in one area might inform another. The goal of the American Psychological Association's (APA's) Clinical Health Psychology series is to change these trends and provide a comprehensive yet concise overview of the essential elements of clinical practice in specific areas of health care. The future of 21st-century health psychology depends on the ability of new practitioners to be innovative and to generalize their knowledge across domains. To this end, the series focuses on a variety of topics and provides a foundation as well as specific clinical examples for mental health professionals who are new to the field.

Working with Susan Reynolds, senior acquisitions editor at APA Books, I am very proud to have had the opportunity to edit this book series. We have chosen authors who are recognized experts in the field and are rethinking the practice of health psychology to be aligned with modern drivers of health care, such as population health, cost of care, quality of care, and the patient experience.

It is difficult to imagine an experience more psychologically challenging than the inability to breathe. Chronic respiratory disease is the third leading cause of death in the United States, yet few mental health professionals receive training in this area. *Psychological Treatment of Patients With Chronic Respiratory Disease*, by Susan M. Labott, addresses a topic long neglected in the clinical health psychology literature. This well-written, concise volume is essential for the practicing clinical health psychologist as well as for any health care provider with an interest in psychological intervention in the context of respiratory disease. The author describes the nature of chronic lung disease and its medical treatments in the first part of the book and succeeds in making the material accessible for readers unfamiliar with the topic. Evidence-based approaches to addressing psychological problems such as depression, anxiety, poor adherence, and end of life are covered in the latter half of the book. Labott is adept at providing case vignettes that effectively illustrate the key concepts. This volume addresses a critical gap in the literature and provides a comprehensive overview of an understudied topic. We are proud to include *Psychological Treatment of Patients With Chronic Respiratory Disease* as part of APA Books' Clinical Health Psychology series!

—*Ellen A. Dornelas, PhD*
Series Editor

Acknowledgments

Thanks to the many patients who shared their challenges, and to the physicians who collaborated in our understanding of the role of psychological factors in pulmonary disease. Thanks also to my parents, Arlene and Robert Labott, for all your support on the journey.

Psychological Treatment of
**Patients With Chronic
Respiratory Disease**

INTRODUCTION

Chronic obstructive pulmonary disease (COPD) has been diagnosed in more than 170 million people worldwide, and asthma occurs in more than 350 million (GBD 2015 Chronic Respiratory Disease Collaborators, 2017). Millions of people die from these diseases each year, often after many years of struggling with shortness of breath, fears about what the future holds, and limitations on their physical activities. Psychological issues (e.g., anxiety, depression, problems with adjustment) associated with chronic pulmonary disease can result in referrals for psychological evaluation and/or intervention. Yet, most mental health professionals have no specific training in how to apply their skills to this population, and there are no books to aid clinicians in addressing the variety of psychological concerns presented by this group.

The purpose of this book is to provide basic medical information about chronic pulmonary disease and about the psychological treatment of pulmonary patients for psychologists and other mental health professionals who have minimal experience working with this group. Clinicians who have not treated patients with pulmonary disease may ask: What is this disease? What is its impact on this person's life? As a treating psychologist, should

http://dx.doi.org/10.1037/0000189-001
Psychological Treatment of Patients With Chronic Respiratory Disease, by S. M. Labott

I do anything differently with this patient than with anyone else? These are the types of questions addressed herein.

The focus is on adults with pulmonary disease and on those chronic respiratory diseases most commonly seen for evaluation and treatment in an outpatient psychology setting, although the information provided here is also relevant for clinicians working as an inpatient or outpatient consultant or as a member of a pulmonary or primary care treatment team. A basic summary of several of the most common chronic respiratory diseases is presented to allow readers to understand medical issues that can affect the patient's psychological state; readers can generalize this knowledge to less common respiratory diseases, when appropriate. Acute pulmonary diseases are not the focus; relative to the chronic and progressive diseases, they present different challenges for patients and are less likely to be seen in the outpatient setting.

Part I provides medical background as context. Chapter 1 describes how the respiratory system works, symptoms of dysfunction, and the typical features of the most common chronic respiratory diseases (i.e., COPD, asthma, fibrosis and pneumoconiosis, pulmonary arterial hypertension, sarcoidosis, cystic fibrosis, sleep apnea). Chapter 2 describes the medical interview, physical examination, and diagnostic testing used to make a diagnosis, as well as the medical treatments for pulmonary diseases. Environmental and occupational exposures that can cause or exacerbate pulmonary diseases are reviewed in Chapter 3, along with information on social influences and genetics.

Part II is focused on the psychological evaluation and treatment of pulmonary patients. Specifically, Chapter 4 describes the steps involved in performing a thorough biopsychosocial evaluation. Adjustment challenges are described in Chapter 5, along with interventions to improve adjustment and factors that affect it. Chapters 6 and 7 describe the prevalence, impacts, and causes of anxiety (Chapter 6) and depression (Chapter 7) in pulmonary patients. Interventions such as psychoeducation, cognitive and behavioral treatments, and psychotropic medication are described for both anxiety and depression. Because smoking tobacco is one of the main causes of pulmonary disease, tobacco and other inhaled substances are discussed in Chapter 8. Assessment, brief interventions, and smoking cessation interventions, such as nicotine replacement, pharmacotherapy, and psychological treatment, are described. Chapter 9 focuses on the impact of chronic respiratory disease on the family and on social support. End-of-life issues are addressed in Chapter 10, including a discussion of withholding or withdrawing life-sustaining treatment, respiratory patients' concerns at the end of their lives, and relevant psychological interventions. Chapter 11 presents ethical and professional issues, including confidentiality, competence, and diversity.

This book is based on the biopsychosocial model, in which relevant biological, psychological, and social factors are integrated to provide a holistic conceptualization of the patient in his environment. This integrative approach is highlighted in both the evaluation and treatment of respiratory patients. The cases provided to illustrate concepts are based on real patients, with identifying information altered to protect their privacy. Throughout the book, providers and patients are referred to as either female or male, to avoid the use of "he/she." Finally, the words *respiratory* and *pulmonary* are used interchangeably.

Patients with chronic pulmonary disease can benefit from psychological treatment, yet many clinicians have little experience or knowledge to inform their work with these patients. This book provides a foundation of knowledge on which to build.

PART **I** OVERVIEW OF
CHRONIC RESPIRATORY
DISEASE IN ADULTS

1 UNDERSTANDING THE RESPIRATORY SYSTEM AND CHRONIC RESPIRATORY DISEASES

Breathing, or *respiration*, moves oxygen (O_2) from outside the body to internal bodily cells and removes carbon dioxide (CO_2) waste. *Inspiration* occurs when the *diaphragm*, a muscle beneath the lungs, contracts. This enlarges the chest cavity, creating a partial vacuum; therefore, intrathoracic pressure is less than air pressure. Air then rushes in from outside the body until the pressure is equalized (see Figure 1.1). *Expiration* is a passive process that occurs when the diaphragm relaxes and abdominal organs move upward, pushing air out of the lungs. The efficiency of this process depends on lung elasticity, known as *compliance.*

During inspiration, air enters the nose (also called *nares*), where it is warmed and moistened, and hair cells (*cilia*) trap foreign particles that could be harmful. The *pharynx* carries food and air, then divides into a separate passageway for each. Air continues through the airway, passing through the *epiglottis*, a flap that closes when an individual swallows to keep foreign materials out of the airway. The larynx contains the *vocal cords* (the voice box), which vibrate to produce sound.

The *trachea* (windpipe) is a rigid tube that is lined with cilia to keep unwanted materials from entering the lungs. It subdivides into *bronchi*,

http://dx.doi.org/10.1037/0000189-002
Psychological Treatment of Patients With Chronic Respiratory Disease, by S. M. Labott

FIGURE 1.1. The Respiratory System

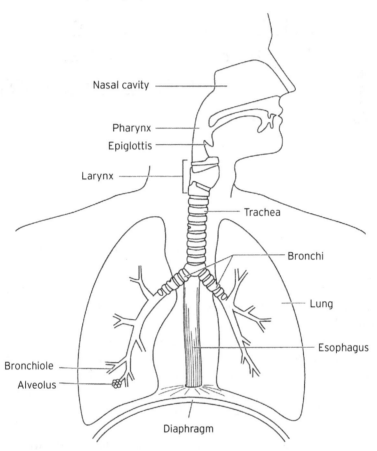

From *Clinical Handbook of Health Psychology* (2nd ed., p. 59), by P. M. Camic and S. J. Knight (Eds.), 2004, Cambridge, MA: Hogrefe & Huber Publishers. Copyright 2004 by Hogrefe & Huber Publishers. Reprinted with permission.

the air passages into the lungs. The bronchi branch into smaller passages (*bronchioles*), ultimately connecting to *alveoli,* which are groupings of air sacks that pass air into the red blood cells (*hemoglobin*) to be circulated through the body. Each lung contains 300 million to 400 million alveoli (Jones, 2017).

Respiration is an involuntary process regulated in the *medulla* (the lowest part of the brainstem). Changes in breathing rate and depth occur in response to changes in elements such as pH (alkalinity/acidity), blood oxygen, CO_2, blood pressure, body temperature, and lung inflation. A normal respiration rate is 12 to 18 breaths per minute. Breathing typically utilizes very little energy, known as *work of breathing*. For individuals with lung disease, however, the work of breathing can increase dramatically; it can take a significant amount of energy if the individual is struggling against narrowed airways to move air in and out of the lungs.

Exercise, medication, emotion, and other factors can impact respiration through the physiological changes associated with them. Individuals can also override the body's natural process, for example, if they hold their breath or intentionally hyperventilate. (See Weinberger, Cockrill, & Mandel, 2019, for more detail on all aspects of the process of respiration.)

RESPIRATORY DISEASES

Lung diseases can be categorized into those involving obstruction, restriction, vascular changes, malignancy, or infection; Exhibit 1.1 lists some common respiratory diseases in each of these categories. The respiratory functions that can be affected by these diseases include ventilation, pulmonary circulation, and gas exchange. *Ventilation* is the successful movement of air from outside the body to the alveoli; this process is impaired in restrictive and obstructive pulmonary diseases. *Pulmonary circulation* involves the movement of blood from the lungs to the heart and back; this can be impaired due to pulmonary hypertension or pulmonary emboli (PE). *Gas exchange* is the removal of CO_2 from the body and the delivery of O_2. (See Kasper et al., 2016, for more detail on these processes.)

Dysfunction anywhere in the respiratory system can result in problems with ventilation, pulmonary circulation, and gas exchange. Specifically, problems can occur with the (a) airway, for example, asthma, chronic obstructive pulmonary disease (COPD), and cystic fibrosis (CF); (b) alveoli, for example, pneumonia, tuberculosis, and acute respiratory distress syndrome; (c) *interstitium* (the lining between alveoli), for example, sarcoidosis and pulmonary fibrosis; (d) blood vessels, for example, PE and pulmonary hypertension; (e) *pleura* (the lining around the lungs), for example, pleural effusion and pneumothorax; or (f) chest wall, for example, amyotrophic lateral sclerosis and myasthenia gravis (WebMD, n.d.-b). Dysfunction in the respiratory system results in symptoms such as cough, dyspnea (shortness of breath), gasping, wheezing, chest pain, and fatigue.

Pulmonary diseases can also be classified as either acute or chronic. Acute disorders are time-limited and can generally be treated and resolved. Chronic disorders can be treated and managed but can generally *not* be

EXHIBIT 1.1. Common Respiratory Diseases by Diagnostic Categories

Obstructive	
Asthma	Cystic fibrosis
Chronic obstructive pulmonary disease	Bronchiolitis
Bronchiectasis	

Restrictive–parenchymal[a]	
Sarcoidosis	Drug- or radiation-induced interstitial
Idiopathic pulmonary fibrosis	lung disease
Desquamative interstitial pneumonitis	Asbestosis
Pneumoconiosis	

Restrictive–extraparenchymal[a]	
Neuromuscular	Chest wall/Pleural disease
Diaphragmatic weakness/paralysis	Kyphoscoliosis
Myasthenia gravis	Obesity
Guillain-Barré syndrome	Ankylosing spondylitis
Muscular dystrophies	Chronic pleural effusions
Cervical spine injury	
Amyotrophic lateral sclerosis	

Pulmonary vascular disease	
Pulmonary embolism	Pulmonary arterial hypertension

Malignancy	
Bronchogenic carcinoma	Cancer metastatic to lung
(small cell or non-small-cell)	

Infectious diseases	
Pneumonia	Bronchitis
Tracheitis	

Note. From *Harrison's Manual of Medicine* (19th ed., p. 706), by D. L. Kasper, A. S. Fauci, S. L. Hauser, D. L. Longo, J. Jameson, and J. Loscalzo (Eds.), 2016, New York, NY: McGraw-Hill. Copyright 2016 by McGraw-Hill Education. Reprinted with permission.
[a]Parenchymal diseases affect the functional lung tissue, whereas extraparenchymal diseases are associated with connective and supporting tissue.

cured, and they may also involve progressive impairment and worsening symptoms over time. Some chronic disorders may also have acute exacerbations, such as COPD and asthma.

The psychological experience of chronic respiratory diseases is often dramatically different from the acute disease experience. Because an acute disorder is generally temporary, a patient's concern about symptoms and associated limitations may be significantly less than that associated with a chronic disorder (e.g., an acute episode of pneumonia); even if an acute disorder results in a hospital admission, it is a different emotional experience than receiving a diagnosis of chronic respiratory disease that will affect the remainder of one's life. Chronic disorders involve ongoing emotional and physical adjustment, greater limitations, and perhaps significant life changes for the patient. With few exceptions, most chronic lung diseases begin in midlife and progress as the patient ages (due to repeated exposures to noxious substances or infection). At early stages, the disease is often undiagnosed, but as it worsens and is associated with greater impairment, the diagnosis is likely to be made. Those patients who are most likely to be seen by an outpatient psychologist are older patients who are experiencing significant impacts on their quality of life due to the chronic lung disease. For this reason, the focus in this book will be on chronic lung disease.

Chronic Obstructive Pulmonary Disease

COPD is "a common, preventable and treatable disease that is characterized by persistent respiratory symptoms and airflow limitation that is due to airway and/or alveolar abnormalities usually caused by significant exposure to noxious particles or gases" (Global Initiative for Chronic Obstructive Lung Disease [GOLD], 2018, p. 4). COPD is the most common category of chronic lung diseases and includes disorders such as emphysema and chronic bronchitis. The prevalence of COPD in 2015 was 174.5 million worldwide, and 3 million people died from it (GBD 2015 Chronic Respiratory Disease Collaborators, 2017). In the United States, 16 million people have been diagnosed with COPD, and millions of others have COPD but have not yet been diagnosed; it is also the fourth main cause of disability in the United States (U.S. Department of Health & Human Services, 2018).

The most common symptoms associated with COPD include dyspnea, cough, and sputum production; patients may also experience wheezing, chest tightness, and congestion (Miravitlles & Ribera, 2017). It is a chronic and progressive disease that affects airflow and results in difficulty breathing. Symptoms gradually worsen over time but not at the same rate for all patients. The disease progression is often marked by exacerbations (periods of acute increases in symptoms) that may require hospitalization.

The primary cause of COPD is tobacco smoke (either active smoking or passive exposure), but individuals without exposure can also develop COPD because other factors can affect the development and course of COPD. *Alpha-1 antitrypsin deficiency*, for example, is a genetic factor that increases the risk of development of COPD. Other physiological and environmental risk factors include age; decreased lung growth in childhood; occupational exposures to dusts, chemicals, and fumes; indoor air pollution; and a history of asthma (see GOLD, 2018, for more detail on each of these). Exacerbations may be precipitated by a new infection, exposure to pollution, bronchospasm (constriction of the bronchiole walls), and heart failure, although the precipitating cause of a COPD exacerbation is not always identifiable (Weinberger et al., 2019).

Asthma

The Global Initiative for Asthma (GINA; 2018) defines *asthma* as "a heterogeneous disease, usually characterized by chronic airway inflammation. It is defined by the history of respiratory symptoms such as wheeze, shortness of breath, chest tightness and cough that vary over time and in intensity, together with variable expiratory airflow limitation" (p. 14). Airway inflammation swells the airways and the surrounding muscles become tight, narrowing the airway and decreasing the amount of air that can flow through it (National Heart, Lung, and Blood Institute, n.d.). Patients with asthma may have periods of no symptoms whatsoever, with intermittent exacerbations. Episodes occur in response to allergies, exercise, infections, irritants, weather changes, and other factors (GINA, 2018). *Status asthmaticus* refers to an extreme episode of asthma that is not responsive to the typical treatments; this can result in hospitalization and may be life-threatening.

The prevalence of asthma in 2015 was 358.2 million people worldwide (GBD 2015 Chronic Respiratory Disease Collaborators, 2017). Asthma can begin in childhood and may continue into adulthood; adult-onset asthma also occurs. About 19 million adults in the United States have asthma (Centers for Disease Control and Prevention, 2019a). Asthma is more common in men but more severe in women, and prevalence is 3 times higher in African Americans who live in urban areas (Myers & Op't Holt, 2016).

Asthma is categorized in terms of its severity and the extent to which it is controlled by treatment. Assessments of both severity and control are based on the patient's level of impairment and future risk. Asthma severity is categorized as *intermittent* (≤ 2 days' symptoms/week), *mild persistent* (> 2 days' symptoms/week), *moderate persistent* (daily symptoms), or *severe persistent* (symptoms occur throughout each day; see Corder, 2017). Asthma control is categorized as *well-controlled, not well-controlled,* or *very poorly controlled,* depending on the symptoms demonstrated, and treatment is adjusted on the basis of these determinations (Myers & Op't Holt, 2016).

Pulmonary Fibrosis

Pulmonary fibrosis refers to a class of lung diseases that are associated with *fibrosis,* the development of connective tissue or scarring after injury. The fibrosis makes breathing difficult because the thickened tissue makes it harder for air to move from alveoli to the blood; symptoms of fibrosis include cough, fatigue, dyspnea, weight loss, and body aches (Mayo Clinic, n.d.).

Causes of pulmonary fibrosis include the inhalation of dusts (see pneumoconiosis in next paragraph), medication and radiation treatments, and other medical conditions (such as systemic lupus erythematosus and rheumatoid arthritis; Pulmonary Fibrosis Foundation, 2019). Pulmonary fibrosis with an unknown cause is known as *idiopathic pulmonary fibrosis* (IPF).

Pneumoconiosis is a type of fibrosis caused by the inhalation and accumulation of dust in the lungs. There are many types of pneumoconiosis, named for the type of dust inhaled, for example, *silicosis* from crystalline silica, *coal workers' pneumoconiosis* (CWP) or *black lung* due to coal dust, and *asbestosis* from asbestos. These diseases can be prevented with adequate dust control (Jones, 2017). They develop and progress over time with repeated and chronic exposure to the dust, often in the context of the patient's occupation. The prevalence of various types of pulmonary fibrosis varies, with IPF affecting about 100,000 people in the United States (National Institutes of Health, U.S. National Library of Medicine, 2019), while over 10% of miners with 25 years of work have CWP (Blackley, Halldin, & Laney, 2018).

Cystic Fibrosis

CF is an autosomal recessive genetic disease (Volsko, O'Malley, & Rubin, 2016) and the most common monogenetic disease in Caucasians (Rowe, Hoover, & Solomon, 2016). It is usually diagnosed in childhood and is a fatal chronic disease, although many patients now live into their 30s and beyond (Mayo Clinic, 2016). More than 30,000 people in the United States are diagnosed with CF (WebMD, n.d.-a). In CF, the body is not able to effectively transfer water and salt in and out of cells, and body fluids (e.g., mucus, sweat, digestive juices) become sticky. The build-up of sticky mucus can cause problems throughout the body, including lung infections, the development of fibrous tissue in the pancreas, and digestive and liver problems; infertility is also common (Priestley, Green, & Abel, 2017). Respiration and digestion are the most common processes affected in CF (Jones, 2017). Pulmonary symptoms include cough, repeated lung infections, wheezing, and shortness of breath; digestive problems include poor absorption of nutrients, malnutrition, and poor growth (Cystic Fibrosis Foundation, n.d.-a).

Pulmonary Hypertension

An increase in blood pressure in the arteries that connect the lungs to the heart is known as pulmonary hypertension (PH). PH reduces blood flow through the arteries and is a chronic and progressive disease. There are five categories of PH, based on its cause: (a) pulmonary arterial hypertension, (b) PH caused by heart disease, (c) PH caused by lung disease, (d) PH caused by chronic blood clots, and (e) PH associated with other conditions (Chin & Channick, 2016; Mayo Clinic, 2017). Regardless of the cause, PH results from changes in the pulmonary arteries that restrict blood flow due to the increased pressure (Jones, 2017).

Overall prevalence of PH is difficult to determine because of the variety of etiologies, but in Europe and the United States, prevalence has been reported at 6.6 to 26 cases per million. Rates vary significantly, depending on other associated diseases, for example, 0.46% has been reported in patients with HIV, but up to 60% in scleroderma (hardening of skin and connective tissue) patients (Medscape, 2018).

As with some other chronic lung diseases, the most significant symptom of PH is dyspnea, which becomes worse with less exertion over time (Chin & Channick, 2016). Other symptoms include fatigue, dizziness, chest pain, swelling, cyanosis (blue lips due to decreased oxygenation), and changes in heart rate or rhythm (Mayo Clinic, 2017).

Sarcoidosis

Sarcoidosis is "an idiopathic, systemic disease in which granuloma formation is pathologically triggered in a susceptible individual" (Landsberg, 2018, p. 179). Sarcoidosis is due to the collection of *granulomas* (clumps of macrophages), but the cause of their development is unknown. The granulomas create inflammation and impair lung function, resulting in cough, dyspnea, and fatigue. Any organ system can be affected, but 95% of patients have pulmonary involvement (Judson, Morgenthau, & Baughman, 2016). Sarcoidosis can be either an acute or chronic disease; chronic sarcoidosis is usually associated with multi-organ involvement such as skin, liver, and eyes (Judson et al., 2016). In the United States, sarcoidosis is most common in those 20 to 40 years old; it occurs more frequently in African Americans than in Whites (Weinberger et al., 2019) and currently affects more than 54,000 people (Health Grades, 2014).

Sleep Apnea

Sleep apnea is a chronic disorder in which people repeatedly stop breathing when sleeping. It is associated with daytime sleepiness, snoring, hypoxemia (low blood oxygen), and disrupted sleep. Although sleep apnea is a breathing problem, it is distinct from the chronic diseases described previously because it is not a dysfunction of the lungs and it does not cause the typical symptoms of chronic lung disease, such as dyspnea or cough. *Obstructive sleep apnea* (OSA) occurs when the pharynx closes, creating an upper airway obstruction during sleep, and the person continues to try to breathe (often gasping); *central* sleep apnea is an abnormality in the brainstem that regulates breathing, and there is no effort to continue breathing (Chaudhary, Taft, & Mishoe, 2016; Cowie, 2017).

OSA is the most common, occurring in 50 million to 70 million adults in the United States (American Sleep Association [ASA], 2019). It is more common in men, and its prevalence increases with obesity and age (ASA, 2019; Chaudhary et al., 2016). If treated properly, generally with continuous positive airway pressure (CPAP), it may have little impact on a patient's daily functioning. Prior to diagnosis, or if the problem is untreated, people endure significant sleepiness, insomnia, headache, and cognitive symptoms.

THE EXPERIENCE OF CHRONIC LUNG DISEASE

"If you can't breathe, nothing else matters" is a slogan that has been used by the American Lung Association (n.d.) to highlight the significant impacts that breathlessness can have on the life of an individual with chronic lung disease. Generally, dyspnea occurs with exertion, and breathlessness becomes worse with less exertion over time. Patients often describe the experience as like breathing through a straw. Although initially this may mean that the individual can no longer engage in intense physical activity comfortably, in later stages she may be unable to perform simple activities of daily living (ADLs), such as eating, bathing, and toileting. People who are unable to exert much control over the symptoms may experience more stress associated with the disease than those who are able to exert more control. Although decreases in physical activity can help to minimize the experience of dyspnea, they may also result in negative effects, such as decreased social interaction, poorer quality of life, and faster disease progression.

As the lung disease progresses, people may need to commit a significant amount of time each day simply to managing their symptoms (e.g., taking medication, attending pulmonary rehabilitation). Patients may also need to adjust to the use of additional aids, such as canes and wheelchairs. *Hypoxia* (decreased oxygen in body tissue), which can result in neuropsychological changes, will need to be managed, often through the use of a ventilator or supplemental oxygen. Chronic lung disease also increases the risk of developing other diseases, such as heart disease and lung cancer (Kohli, 2016).

People may experience guilt if they believe they created the disease themselves, through their own behavior (e.g., smoking). Patients may experience anxiety due to shortness of breath, and they may also become depressed due to the limitations on their lives. Young adults with CF will likely die at a much younger age than their peers; that knowledge can have a significant impact on their life choices and emotional state throughout their lives. Issues associated with adjustment, anxiety, and depression in chronic lung disease, as well as psychological interventions to address these challenges, are discussed in detail in later chapters.

2 DIAGNOSIS AND TREATMENT OF PULMONARY DISEASE

An accurate diagnosis of a specific respiratory disease requires the integration of data from a clinical interview, a physical examination, and diagnostic testing. The diagnostic workup can create anxiety for many patients because the examinations and procedures are often foreign to them. Information about these procedures can help patients to develop realistic expectations and may decrease anxiety.

CLINICAL INTERVIEW

The clinical interview, performed by the patient's doctor or her surrogate, begins with a patient's description of her chief complaint and her health history. The pulmonologist will ask about the symptoms the patient is experiencing to elicit information on their onset, location, duration, quality and quantity, the setting in which they occur, factors that alleviate or trigger them, and treatments that relieve or intensify the symptoms. The symptoms generally most relevant to the diagnosis of pulmonary disease include dyspnea (shortness of breath), cough, wheezing, and sputum production.

http://dx.doi.org/10.1037/0000189-003
Psychological Treatment of Patients With Chronic Respiratory Disease, by S. M. Labott

During the initial clinical interview, patients are also asked about their work history and travel to determine exposures to toxins or other factors associated with lung disease. The patient's daily activities are discussed to assess any limitations on physical activity as well as changes in activity. Smoking history and the patient's medical history and that of his family are obtained. A review of systems then provides data on any other physical problems that the patient has throughout the body. For patients who have not yet participated in the medical interview, it is helpful to have them consider the questions they will be asked and make notes regarding specific details about their symptoms. Curtis (2017) and Simmons (2016) provided more extensive descriptions of the information to be obtained from the patient during the medical interview.

PHYSICAL EXAM

The examiner will attend to the rate, depth, and pattern of respiration, as well as skin color and chest characteristics. She will feel the body for masses, movement, and other characteristics (*palpation*). *Chest percussion* involves the examiner placing a finger against a body part, then tapping it with a finger from the opposite hand. Percussion produces sounds that provide diagnostic data (i.e., different tones are associated with normal vs. abnormal structures). *Auscultation* involves listening to the lungs and breathing with a stethoscope to assess for abnormalities. With training, examiners learn to differentiate normal versus abnormal breathing sounds. Abnormal breathing sounds include crackles (popping sounds that signify problems with small airways), rhonchi (rumbling sounds due to secretions), wheezes and stridor (whistles due to airway narrowing; called either a *wheeze* or *stridor* based on location), and friction rubs (a rasping sound caused by the lungs and chest wall rubbing each other, often due to inflammation). The physician will also check for *clubbing* (fingernails that curve down and over the skin), which is a characteristic associated with certain lung diseases. The physical exam itself should cause no pain or discomfort for patients. Curtis (2017), Simmons (2016), and Weinberger et al. (2019) offer more detail on the physical examination.

DIAGNOSTIC TESTING

Many and varied diagnostic tests are available to aid in the diagnosis of lung disease. Some of the more common tests are briefly described in this section.

Pulmonary Function Testing

Pulmonary function tests (PFTs) are performed using a *spirometer*, equipment that measures aspects of lung functioning as the patient breathes through a tube that is connected to it. (PFTs are sometimes also referred to as *spirometry*.) Patients initially breathe normally into the tube, and then they perform a specific breathing maneuver in which they fill their lungs with as much air as possible, then exhale as quickly and forcefully as possible, then continue to expel all the air from the lungs. The maneuver is performed several times, but accurate results are obtained only if the patient does the maneuver properly and with maximum effort. There is no pain associated with this testing, although some patients have difficulty performing the maneuver and exerting maximal effort when doing so.

PFT results provide data on lung volume (the capacity of the lungs), flow rates (airflow in the airways), and diffusing capacity (ease of gas transfer; Weinberger et al., 2019). PFTs are critical to the diagnosis of many pulmonary diseases, can help to determine if the patient has an obstructive or restrictive lung disease, and can assess disease severity. Exhibit 2.1 contains a list of some of the most important values obtained from pulmonary function testing and their meaning. A patient's values are compared with normative values based on age, gender, height, and ethnicity. Haynes (2016) included more details on PFTs and the interpretation of results.

Peak flow can also be measured with a simple handheld device. Patients with asthma are often taught to use a portable peak flow meter to assess their symptoms to decide if they need to use a rescue inhaler or take other medication to prevent an attack.

EXHIBIT 2.1. Common Pulmonary Function Tests and Their Meanings

FEV_1: forced expiratory volume in 1 second; volume of air expired in 1st second during maneuver
VC: vital capacity; total air volume exhaled after maximum inspiration
$FEF_{25\%-75\%}$: forced expiratory flow from 25% to 75% of exhale
FRC: functional residual capacity; air volume remaining in lungs after normal exhale
FVC: forced vital capacity; amount of air exhaled forcefully after maximum inhale
SVC: slow vital capacity; same as VC, but slow and total
RV: residual volume; amount of air remaining in lungs after complete expiration
TLC: total lung capacity; RV + SVC = maximum inspiration
VT: tidal volume; amount of air exhaled during normal breathing
MV: minute volume; amount of air breathed each minute
IRV: inspiratory reserve volume; amount of air that can be inhaled beyond normal inspiration
ERV: expiratory reserve volume; amount of air that can be exhaled beyond tidal volume
PEFR: peak expiratory flow rate; maximal expiratory flow with maximum patient effort

Body Plethysmography

Performed in a pulmonary function laboratory, this testing measures lung volumes and airway resistance and conductance. Patients sit inside an airtight rectangular plastic booth (which looks like an old telephone booth) and breathe into a tube. Pressure changes within the box result in associated changes in lung volume. Plethysmography can quickly and accurately provide information on absolute air volumes in the lungs. There is no discomfort associated with this procedure, and because the booth is clear, patients are generally not claustrophobic.

Diffusing Capacity

This test measures the rate of transfer of air from the alveoli to the blood. In a pulmonary function laboratory, patients breathe in a small amount of carbon monoxide, hold it briefly, then blow it out quickly. Diffusing capacity of carbon monoxide (DLCO) is measured, providing an approximation of oxygen diffusion. The patient's results are compared with norms based on gender, age, height, and ethnicity. DLCO results can be interpreted as a percentage of the predicted value, with at least 80% predicted considered to be normal. They can also be interpreted in relation to the lower limit of normal (LLN). A result above the LLN is considered normal, and results below the LLN are rated in terms of severity.

Arterial Blood Gases

Obtained from a sample of blood drawn from a radial artery (a branch of the brachial artery that passes from the elbow, through the wrist and palm, and finally into the fingers), arterial blood gases (ABGs) are often performed in the inpatient hospital setting. From the patient's perspective, the collection of the sample for ABGs is similar to a blood draw. ABGs provide data on gas exchange from measurements of partial pressure of oxygen, partial pressure of carbon dioxide, and pH (a measure of alkalinity or acidity). These values are considered together to determine problems with carbon dioxide removal, blood oxygen content, and acid-base balance (for more detail, see Weinberger et al., 2019).

Pulse Oximetry

This procedure provides a measure of the oxygen saturation of hemoglobin (O_2 sat). It is done by attaching a clip to the patient's finger that passes light through the finger; oxygenated and deoxygenated hemoglobin have different absorption rates, so the saturation can be measured (Weinberger et al., 2019). Normal O_2 sat is 95% to 100%; abnormally low saturation is called *hypoxemia*. Decreased saturation may result in impairments in cognitive functioning and can affect organ functioning throughout the body. Pulse oximetry may be used instead of ABGs because it is much simpler and less intrusive, although it provides less information than that obtained from ABGs.

Bronchoscopy

This is a procedure in which a tube is guided through the nose or mouth (which is numbed) down into the airway. The bronchoscope is fitted with a camera, and images of the airway are viewed on a monitor. Bronchoscopy may be done either as an inpatient or outpatient procedure, depending on the specific method employed (which dictates the associated risk). Samples can be taken from the airway: in a procedure called *bronchoalveolar lavage*, saline is ejected into the alveolar spaces and samples are collected; lung biopsies and needle aspiration can extract cell samples for further analysis.

Patients lay on a table in a procedure room for the bronchoscopy. The nose/mouth area is anesthetized so there is no pain, and patients are minimally sedated so that they are aware during the procedure but are comfortable; they typically do not recall it later. Patients do not usually like the idea of a tube going into their lungs, but they generally tolerate it well. Bleeding is the most common risk but is only of major concern for those with clotting disorders or on anticoagulant medications.

Bronchoscopy is most often performed when patients report hemoptysis (coughing up blood) or when there is concern for an infection or cancer. In many cases, a visual inspection of the airway or an analysis of cell samples can confirm a diagnosis.

Provocation Testing

Often referred to as a "challenge," this is a procedure that is done in a pulmonary function laboratory, usually if there is a question of asthma. Because symptoms may not be present when the patient is in the physician's office, provocation testing involves the patient inhaling a substance to determine how the airway responds. Patients with asthma will demonstrate greater airway responsiveness to the challenge of certain drugs. The most common substance used to perform provocation testing is methacholine, but histamine or mannitol can also be used (Global Initiative for Asthma

[GINA], 2018). Patients are often fearful that the challenge will bring on a serious asthma attack. They may experience some mild symptoms, but the test is stopped before any significant symptoms or discomfort occur.

Chest Radiographs (X-Rays) and Computed Tomography

X-rays are commonly used in evaluating lung disease because structures can be easily seen and abnormalities identified on the X-ray. A computed tomography scan provides additional cross-sectional detail but is more expensive and exposes the patient to more radiation. Both procedures are non-invasive and only require the patient to remain still while the images are recorded (see Weinberger et al., 2019, for more detail on these procedures).

Skin Prick Tests

These are performed to determine if specific antigens (foreign substances that elicit an immune response) are associated with asthma symptoms. Allergens (substances that can elicit an allergic reaction) are placed underneath the skin (along with control substances). Skin reactivity can be measured to determine whether the person is allergic to any of the substances tested (e.g., Doe, 2017).

Sweat Test

Used to diagnose cystic fibrosis (CF), pilocarpine is placed on the arm and a small amount of electrical stimulation is applied for a few minutes. This makes the person sweat. Patients may feel some tingling, but there is no pain. The sweat is collected for 30 minutes, and the amount of chloride it contains is measured (Cystic Fibrosis Foundation, n.d.-b). People with CF demonstrate higher levels of chloride in their sweat. For most adult patients, this test was completed in childhood when the diagnosis of CF was initially made.

Six Minute Walk Test (6MWT)

In this test, patients walk on a level surface for 6 minutes. The distance walked and the O_2 saturation during the walk provide data on the patient's functional ability to exercise, although the 6MWT provides no information on the cause of an exercise limitation. Older patients, those with significant lung disease, and those who are deconditioned may find a 6 minute walk difficult to perform.

Polysomnography

Often referred to as a "sleep study," a polysomnogram records EEG (brain waves), EKG (heart rate and rhythm), EMG (muscle activity), as well as possible additional measures while the individual sleeps. Apneas (cessation of airflow for 10+ seconds) and hypopneas (airflow decreased by at least 30%) can be documented and counted. The number of these events that occur while the individual sleeps determines the presence and severity of obstructive sleep apnea (OSA) and dictates the appropriate treatment. In conjunction with the polysomnography, patients may be given questionnaires to assess their subjective experience; for example, the Epworth Sleepiness Scale (Johns, 1991) assesses daytime sleepiness if there is a concern about obstructive sleep apnea.

To perform a sleep study, the patient needs to remain overnight in the sleep laboratory, similar to a hospital room. It is common that, once the presence of OSA is confirmed, the patient may be wakened during the night to put on a mask to titrate continuous positive airway pressure (CPAP). CPAP provides pressure in the airway to keep it from closing and is the most common treatment for OSA.

Patients resist sleep studies because of the inconvenience of spending an entire night away from home and also because of the discomfort of wearing the brain, heart, and muscle monitors while trying to sleep, although there is no pain. Many are also anxious about wearing a CPAP mask on the face (discussed in Chapter 6).

INTEGRATING DATA FOR DIAGNOSIS

Table 2.1 provides examples of how combinations of the patient's report of history and symptoms, the physical examination, and diagnostic testing are used to develop a diagnosis for the lung diseases described in Chapter 1. Certain parameters provide evidence for or against a specific diagnosis. In practice, however, the diagnostic process involves significantly more information than that shown here, and the physician's clinical experience is also an important factor.

TREATMENT OF PULMONARY DISEASE

Treatment of chronic lung disease is designed to manage symptoms, improve patient functioning, decrease exacerbations, and slow disease progression. With a few exceptions, there is no cure for chronic lung disease. Exhibit 2.2

TABLE 2.1. Examples of Interview, Exam, and Testing Data for Sample Chronic Lung Diseases

Chronic lung disease	Clinical interview	Physical exam	Diagnostic testing
COPD	History of chronic dyspnea and cough; smoking	Hyperresonant chest sounds; prolonged expiration	X-ray shows hyper-inflation; FEV_1/VC ratio demonstrates airflow obstruction; DLCO reduced
Asthma	History of episodes of wheezing and coughing	Wheezing heard during expiration	Airway narrowing with methacholine challenge; FEV_1 and FVC show reversible airflow obstruction
Pulmonary fibrosis[a]	Dyspnea, fatigue, weight loss	Crackles; clubbing	TLC decreased, i.e., restriction; DLCO reduced
Cystic fibrosis	History of bronchial infections in childhood	Wheezing, crackles, rhonchi	Elevated chloride on sweat test
Pulmonary hypertension	Complaints of dyspnea and fatigue	Changes in heart sounds	Pulmonary arteries increased in size on X-ray; redistribution of blood flow; arterial PO_2 decreased
Sarcoidosis	Dyspnea and cough	Eye and skin involvement	Lung volume decreased (e.g., TLC, VC); adenopathy or parenchymal disease on X-ray; FEV_1/FVC is normal
Sleep apnea	Daytime sleepiness; snoring	Hypertension	Sleep study demonstrates apneic events

Note. COPD = chronic obstructive pulmonary disease; FEV_1 = forced expiratory volume in 1 second; VC = vital capacity; DLCO = diffusing capacity of carbon monoxide; FVC = forced vital capacity; TLC = total lung capacity; PO_2 = partial pressure of oxygen.
[a]Includes pneumoconiosis.

outlines some of the major treatments for the chronic lung diseases described in Chapter 1; some of the more common treatments are described later. Case 2.1 describes the evaluation and initial treatment of a patient newly diagnosed with chronic obstructive pulmonary disease (COPD).

Smoking Cessation

The most important treatment for many lung diseases is smoking cessation. Abstinence from smoking will not reverse physiological changes that have

EXHIBIT 2.2. Treatments for Chronic Lung Disease

Chronic obstructive pulmonary disease
   Smoking cessation
   Bronchodilators and inhaled corticosteroids
   Pulmonary rehabilitation
   Supplemental oxygen
   Surgery
   Mechanical ventilation

Asthma
   Inhaled anti-inflammatory, bronchodilator, or combination medication
   Systemic corticosteroids for status asthmaticus
   Allergen avoidance

Pulmonary fibrosis
   Corticosteroids
   Cytotoxic agents
   Lung transplantation

Cystic fibrosis
   Antibiotics for active infection
   Optimize nutritional status
   Chest physiotherapy
   Lung transplantation

Pulmonary hypertension
   Vasodilators, anticoagulant medications
   Heart or heart-lung transplantation
   Treatment of heart disease
   Supplemental oxygen

Sarcoidosis
   No treatment for some patients
   Corticosteroids, immunosuppressive drugs

Sleep apnea
   Continuous positive airway pressure

Note. Data from Gibson and Waters (2017); Short and Ghio (2016); Volsko, O'Malley, and Rubin (2016); Weinberger, Cockrill, and Mandel (2019).

already occurred, but it will typically slow disease progression and improve daily symptoms. There are a variety of methods to achieve abstinence, including nicotine replacement, medication, and psychological treatments. Chapter 8 is dedicated to this topic and includes information on the respiratory effects of smoking as well as detailed descriptions of the many interventions available to aid cessation.

CASE 2.1
NEW DIAGNOSIS OF CHRONIC OBSTRUCTIVE PULMONARY DISEASE

Mr. G is a 62-year-old man who attends a pulmonary clinic after complaining to his internist about breathlessness. The patient describes shortness of breath that has occurred over the past two years and seems to be worsening. He describes a feeling of chest tightness, breathlessness, and coughing when he mows the lawn, hurries to catch a bus, or plays football with his grandson. Thus far, he is still able to do these activities, although he has to slow down to maintain comfortable breathing. Patient denies recent travel. He acknowledges smoking a pack of cigarettes daily for 40 years but notes that he has cut back to a half pack per day in the past six months. He reports being diagnosed with diabetes and hypertension but denies other medical problems.

Mr. G undergoes PFTs, which show airflow obstruction and mild lung hyperinflation. Pulse oximetry and respiratory rate are normal. Physical exam demonstrates hyperresonant chest sounds.

The patient is diagnosed with COPD. He is counseled on the need to quit smoking completely. He agrees and wishes to try nicotine replacement using a patch. He is prescribed a short-acting bronchodilator (via MDI) to use when symptoms occur, and he is trained in the proper use of the inhaler. He is scheduled to return to the pulmonary clinic in two months to evaluate the effect of these prescriptions and to determine if additional medical intervention is needed.

When meeting with the pulmonologist, the patient was observed to be quite anxious, so he was introduced to the mental health practitioner on the treatment team who did a brief evaluation in the pulmonary clinic. The patient reported a history of mild anxiety that increased with the diagnosis of COPD. The psychologist acknowledged the patient's concerns about how his life will change as a result of the diagnosis, and they discussed some brief interventions to help the patient cope. Plans were also made for the psychologist to see the patient for a few additional visits to conduct a more thorough evaluation, to provide anxiety management strategies, and to aid the patient in adjusting to the new illness.

Medication

Medications designed to improve airflow are the mainstay of pharmacological treatments for chronic lung disease. Depending on the specific pulmonary problem, short- or long-acting oral medications may be administered daily. Inhaled medications can be delivered in a variety of different ways, such as through metered dose inhalers (MDIs), dry powder inhalers, or nebulizers. In addition, some medications are administered by injection. The type of medication and the delivery method are determined by specific disease characteristics, the patient's symptoms, and symptom severity. Some medications are prescribed for daily use, whereas others are used only in the context of acute symptoms (e.g., the use of a "rescue inhaler" for acute symptoms).

Bronchodilators

These medications dilate the muscles in the respiratory system to widen the airway and allow air to flow more smoothly. Several classes of medications function as bronchodilators, such as $beta_2$-agonists (e.g., salbutamol, terbutaline), anticholinergics (e.g., ipratropium bromide), muscarinic antagonists (e.g., tiotropium, glycopyrronium), and methylxanthines (e.g., aminophylline, theophylline); patients are often prescribed combination medications (Burns, 2017; Global Initiative for Chronic Obstructive Lung Disease [GOLD], 2018; Kohli, 2016). Bronchodilators can be associated with anxiety symptoms; see Chapter 6.

A patient with COPD might take an oral long-acting bronchodilator daily to manage ongoing symptoms; patients with asthma may not take bronchodilators daily but may carry an inhaler containing a short-acting bronchodilator to use in case of an acute episode of asthma. Many patients will take daily medication and also carry an inhaler for quick relief if symptoms become severe.

Anti-Inflammatories

These medications decrease inflammation and narrowing of the airway. This is particularly important in patients with asthma because the airways are hyperresponsive and constrict in response to a variety of stimuli. For this reason, anti-inflammatories are the first line of treatment for asthma (Myers & Op't Holt, 2016).

Corticosteroids are the most commonly used class of anti-inflammatory; the medication can be inhaled daily for asthma control and can also be taken orally or intravenously for quick symptom reduction in emergency situations (Myers & Op't Holt, 2016). In the context of COPD, inhaled corticosteroids are usually combined with long-term bronchodilators to obtain the most benefit (Burns, 2017). Oral glucocorticoids (a type of corticosteroid) are useful in the context of COPD exacerbation, although not usually in daily treatment (GOLD, 2018). For the treatment of sarcoidosis, prednisone (an oral corticosteroid) is the treatment of choice (Jones, 2017).

Corticosteroids can provide many benefits to patients with respiratory disease and other disorders. However, they are associated with a variety of physical side effects, such as osteoporosis, diabetes, cataracts, weakness, and water retention. They are also associated with psychological side effects and can cause symptoms of anxiety, depression, and delirium (*steroid psychosis*). Especially if patients are taking high doses of steroids, the mental health clinician will want to monitor their adherence and help patients to manage any side effects.

Antibiotics

These are used for the treatment of infections. CF is associated with repeated lung infections, so oral and inhaled antibiotics are used frequently, although they are associated with a variety of unwanted side effects such as photosensitivity, nausea, and dizziness (Priestley et al., 2017). Antibiotics are also useful for COPD patients who develop lung infections (Burns, 2017).

Vasodilators

For use in some types of pulmonary hypertension, vasodilators widen blood vessels and reduce vascular resistance, improving blood flow. These medications are often administered through intravenous infusion, but some can be inhaled or taken orally.

Chest Physiotherapy

One of the main problems in CF is the development of thick secretions that are difficult to remove from the airways and that decrease ventilation, creating difficulty breathing. Several techniques have been developed to aid in the removal of the secretions. Chest percussion involves pounding the chest (by either a caretaker or mechanically) to stimulate the patient to cough up secretions. Other methods of chest physiotherapy involve specific breathing techniques or the administration of positive expiratory pressure (applied through a mask). Also useful in COPD, chest wall compression is stimulation delivered through an inflatable vest worn by the patient; the vest pulses to stimulate the movement of airway secretions. Volsko, O'Malley, and Rubin (2016) included more information on chest physiotherapy techniques.

Supplemental Oxygen (O$_2$)

For those with hypoxemia, oxygen is administered through either a mask or nasal cannula. The O$_2$ does not fix the underlying problem but can prevent organ damage due to prolonged hypoxemia. The O_2 may be administered temporarily in an acute situation until the respiratory problem is resolved. Some patients need it only at night or when exerting themselves, whereas others require it continually. Supplemental O_2 is commonly used for patients with severe COPD; portable containers that can be carried in a backpack or attached to walkers and wheelchairs are popular with patients who need to carry it with them at all times. Patients should be made aware that no one should smoke cigarettes near an oxygen tank due to the risk of fire.

Pulmonary Rehabilitation

Pulmonary rehabilitation (PR) describes a multidisciplinary program that provides several different interventions to improve the patient's quality of life and functioning in the context of chronic lung disease. PR programs are quite diverse in terms of the number and type of intervention sessions, as well as the topics covered. Most were developed for COPD treatment, but they can also be useful for other lung diseases. Exercise training and education are generally the main focus. Patients are educated about the pulmonary disease, its effects, and treatments (e.g., proper use of inhalers or medications). They may also learn strategies to manage exacerbations. Because many patients become inactive if they experience dyspnea with exercise, they are also trained in the importance of appropriate exercise techniques. Because less activity will decrease their functional ability, they learn specific exercises that allow them to do more and do it safely. Subjective breathlessness, heart rate, and O_2 saturation may be continually monitored while they exercise.

Patients also learn specific strategies to help them compensate for the pulmonary disease. For example, COPD patients learn pursed-lip breathing in which they breathe in through the nose, then exhale through almost completely closed lips (like blowing one large bubble through a child's soap wand; Custodio, 1998); this improves gas exchange and decreases shortness of breath. Patients may also receive instruction on how to organize home chores (e.g., place most commonly used items on chest level shelves to avoid reaching above their heads) and to pace activities (e.g., work 15 minutes and then rest 15 minutes).

Many PR programs provide patients with psychosocial support. Patients may learn how to cope with feelings of anxiety or depression and how to manage changes in roles and relationships. Although much of the education and exercise is tailored for the specific patient, some of the didactic and social support activities may be done in groups. Patients may attend PR over the long term or they may participate in an intensive program and then continue exercises at home. Many studies have documented positive effects of PR programs on quality of life and exercise capacity (e.g., Puhan, Gimeno-Santos, Cates, & Troosters, 2016) as well as mortality and hospital admissions (e.g., Mukundu & Matiti, 2015). MacIntyre and Crouch (2016) and Tucker and Stoermer (2017) contain more detail on PR.

Mechanical Ventilation

Mechanical ventilation is warranted for patients in acute respiratory failure or for those with chronic respiratory illnesses that make it impossible for them to maintain adequate gas exchange on their own. For those with chronic respiratory illness, the work of breathing may be more than the patient can manage, but mechanical ventilation can provide adequate oxygenation while allowing the respiratory muscles to rest (see Weinberger et al., 2019). In the acute care setting, ventilation may be required temporarily until the patient recovers from an acute injury or illness. Continuous mechanical ventilation may be required in severe cases of COPD, for patients with neuromuscular disease, or for others who are unable to breathe adequately on their own for the long term.

All mechanical ventilation facilitates gas exchange and decreases the work of breathing by controlling either air volume or pressure. The ventilation can be delivered in many different ways, with ventilator settings dictated by the needs of the specific patient. Some common ventilator modes include continuous mandatory ventilation, synchronized intermittent mandatory ventilation, and continuous positive airway pressure (CPAP; commonly used in patients with obstructive sleep apnea). For patients with irreversible respiratory impairments who require continuous ventilation, it is most often delivered through a tracheostomy tube rather than with a tube down the throat (which is more common in the acute care setting). Those who require only intermittent ventilation (often at night) may have it delivered through a mask or mouthpiece.

Surgery

Surgical procedures are indicated for some chronic lung diseases. For example, in severe cases of COPD, surgical procedures such as giant bullectomy and lung volume reduction surgery (LVRS) can provide benefit. Giant bullae are large air spaces in the lungs that are caused by tissue destruction; they compress adjacent healthy tissue. Removal of these is known as bullectomy. LVRS involves the removal of a portion of damaged lung tissue, resulting in improved airflow and less air trapping. However, both LVRS and bullectomy provide benefit for only a subset of COPD patients (Kohli, 2016).

Lung transplantation of either one or both lungs is a treatment option for some patients with severe lung disease. The diseases most associated with lung transplant are COPD, idiopathic pulmonary fibrosis, and CF; 80% of transplant patients have one of these diagnoses (Seneviratne & Hopkins, 2019). As the disease continues to progress while patients are on a waitlist for transplant, the medical symptoms are treated through traditional means, in an effort to keep the patient as functional as possible. Transplantation brings many challenges for patients as they go through a comprehensive evaluation process, wait for an organ to become available, experience the surgical procedure and hospitalization, and then deal with other potential problems such as side effects of medications and organ rejection. Further information about the medical treatment of lung transplant patients can be found in Glanville (2019) and Adegunsoye, Strek, Garrity, Guzy, and Bag (2017); a discussion of the psychological challenges inherent in organ transplantation and relevant interventions can be found in Rainer, Thompson, and Lambros (2010).

CONCLUSION

The workup for the diagnosis of pulmonary disease can be challenging for many patients, often involving a series of examinations and tests that are new to them. Providing information on what these tests involve can help to decrease their concern. Following a diagnosis, the patient should be provided with information on the disease, treatments, and the probable course from the medical team, with explicit information provided on the prescribed treatment regimen. This can be a difficult time for patients because the new diagnosis and treatment details may be overwhelming. The psychologist may need to review the medical information with the patient and can also help the patient with adherence, adjustment, and anxiety or depressive symptoms that may occur (specific interventions are discussed in later chapters).

3

ENVIRONMENTAL, SOCIAL, AND GENETIC INFLUENCES ON CHRONIC RESPIRATORY DISEASE

Many factors can influence the development and/or course of chronic respiratory disease. These factors include occupational and environmental exposures, gender, race and ethnicity, age, behavior, health literacy, and genetics. The impact of these risk factors can be decreased or eliminated by making changes in the social or physical environment.

OCCUPATIONAL AND ENVIRONMENTAL EXPOSURES

Many patients develop chronic respiratory disease secondary to exposure to substances either at work or in the home environment. Much attention is currently focused on prevention and treatment to decrease the impact of these substances.

Workplace Exposures

The inhalation of specific dusts, chemicals, and allergens can result in the development of new lung disease or can exacerbate preexisting lung

http://dx.doi.org/10.1037/0000189-004

disease. It is estimated that 10% to 15% of the burden of chronic obstructive pulmonary disease (COPD) results from occupational exposures to vapors, gases, dusts, and fumes (Fishwick et al., 2015), and 9% to 25% of asthma in adults is caused by occupational exposures (Baur & Bakehe, 2014). Inhaled inorganic dusts, such as silica, asbestos, coal, talc, mica, aluminum, and beryllium, can cause pneumoconiosis (diffuse parenchymal lung disease; Weinberger, Cockrill, & Mandel, 2019). Miners are particularly at risk for inhalation of these dusts. Several factors determine the impact of exposure to these substances. For example, the development of coal workers' pneumoconiosis ("black lung") usually takes many years of exposure for disease development and depends on the type of coal dust inhaled, its concentration, as well as any protective methods used, such as respirators (Ahuja, Kanne, & Meyer, 2015).

Individuals involved in food manufacturing can also develop lung disease as a result of exposures; for example, the butter flavoring diacetyl, used in microwave popcorn, can cause lung disease (Ahuja et al., 2015; Stenton, 2017). Bakers, pastry makers, and other food processors can develop asthma because of exposures to flour, enzymes, and chemicals (Ahuja et al., 2015). Health care workers are exposed to a variety of chemicals, irritants, medications, and latex that are associated with asthma (a long list of specific agents that can cause asthma in health care workers can be found in Mazurek & Weissman, 2016). Inhalation of construction dust has been associated with COPD in construction workers (Borup, Kirkeskov, Hanskov, & Brauer, 2017).

Farmers and landscapers can experience respiratory problems because of exposures to pesticides (e.g., Kearney, Xu, Hight, & Arcury, 2013; Mamane, Baldi, Tessier, Raherison, & Bouvier, 2015), as well as dusts, bacteria, animal dander, and other inhaled substances (e.g., Fontana et al., 2017; Stoleski, Minov, Karadzinska-Bislimovska, & Mijakoski, 2015). Those who work with animals in other settings, such as research laboratories and veterinary clinics, can develop asthma secondary to allergens found in animal products such as hair, saliva, and urine (Stave, 2018).

Many other agents can cause respiratory diseases; in fact, more than 400 agents have been associated with occupational asthma (V. Trivedi, Apala, & Iyer, 2017). These affect numerous occupations in addition to those described previously, including hairdressers, welders, cleaners, spray painters, and those working in maritime environments (Ahuja et al., 2015; Lucas, Lodde, Jepsen, Dewitte, & Jegaden, 2016). Fishwick et al. (2015) provided an extensive list of occupations associated with COPD.

Veterans may also experience respiratory problems due to a military exposure to Agent Orange, one of the herbicides used by the U.S. military during the Vietnam War. Agent Orange has been associated with a wide variety of diseases, including COPD (Yi, Hong, Ohrr, & Yi, 2014; Yi, Ohrr, Hong, & Yi, 2013).

Respiratory disease that is caused by the substances noted previously typically occurs as a result of repeated exposures to the dust or chemical over a significant period of time. Yet, one major exposure over a relatively short period of time can also result in respiratory symptoms and chronic lung disease. Police officers, firefighters, construction workers, and others who were present after the World Trade Center (WTC) attack inhaled significant amounts of dust from concrete, asbestos, and silica, as well as other irritants (e.g., gypsum and calcium carbonate; Ekenga & Friedman-Jiménez, 2011). Many individuals exposed to these substances after the WTC attack developed respiratory diseases such as asthma, COPD, sarcoidosis, and idiopathic pulmonary fibrosis (IPF; e.g., Cleven, Webber, Zeig-Owens, Hena, & Prezant, 2017; Sutherland, Sciurba, Glazer, & Halpern, 2012; Trethewey & Walters, 2018), as well as other physical and mental health problems (e.g., Jordan et al., 2019).

The psychological sequelae of pulmonary disease can include symptoms of anxiety and depression (described in later chapters). These symptoms may be exacerbated if the disease occurred because of an occupational exposure, as workers may be angry that they were exposed to chemicals or dust that made them chronically ill, or stressed by workplace changes or disability procedures. Certain specific exposures may result in additional psychological problems (e.g., PTSD) associated with WTC exposures.

Environmental (Nonoccupational) Exposures

Urban air pollution has long been associated with asthma exacerbations, and there is some evidence that it may result in new cases of asthma as well (Guarnieri & Balmes, 2014). Recent work has also demonstrated the impacts of air pollution on morbidity and mortality in COPD and IPF (DeVries, Kriebel, & Sama, 2017; Sesé et al., 2018). *Environmental tobacco smoke* (often referred to as *secondhand smoke*) has been associated with respiratory disease in adults and is associated with asthma and other problems, including neurocognitive and behavioral effects in children (Reardon, 2007).

Biomass smoke is most common in developing countries in which people burn biomass fuel (e.g., grass, corn, crop residue, fossil coal) for heating and cooking. Inhalation of the smoke can cause *hut lung*, a form of pneumoconiosis (e.g., Seaman, Meyer, & Kanne, 2015).

Treatment and Prevention of Lung Disease Associated With Occupational and Environmental Exposures

The management of exposures can be categorized into (a) primary prevention, prior to disease onset; (b) secondary prevention, which involves detection and occurs early in the disease process; and (c) tertiary prevention, which is the treatment of the disease once it has developed. The intervention strategies focus on education, early detection, avoidance or minimization of exposures, and treatment of disease. Exhibit 3.1 provides examples of interventions at each of these stages.

Note that the intervention strategies are focused on both the individual and on the workplace. That is, workers are educated about healthy procedures and monitoring of their own health, while medical treatment is provided for any existing symptoms or diseases. At the same time, efforts are made to improve the safety of the workplace through changes in the environment and through the use of protective aids. The National Institute for Occupational Safety and Health (NIOSH) provides information on exposures and guidelines to manage them on their website (https://www.cdc.gov/niosh/).

SOCIAL AND DEMOGRAPHIC INFLUENCES

Social variables can play a part in the development and course of chronic pulmonary disease. Some of the social variables are fixed, but others are behavioral and can be changed to improve disease outcomes.

EXHIBIT 3.1. Workplace Prevention Strategies for Occupational Exposures

Primary prevention	Eliminate the use of relevant vapors, gases, dusts, and fumes
	Educate workers about substances and their negative effects
	Train workers to avoid exposure
	Make changes to the environment (e.g., ventilation, temperature) to reduce risk
	Reassign at-risk workers (e.g., those with preexisting respiratory disease)
	Develop and implement legislation to enforce safe practices
Secondary prevention	Medical surveillance, e.g., spirometry
	Monitor worker reports of symptoms
Tertiary prevention	Treatment as usual for respiratory disease
	Prevent further exposure, e.g., consistent use of respirator

Note. Data from Cullinan et al. (2017); Henneberger et al. (2011); Trivedi, Apala, and Iyer (2017).

Gender

Most research on sex differences in chronic respiratory disease has been completed with asthma and COPD patients. Historically, COPD occurred more frequently in men, but since about 2000, the prevalence in men and women is about equal (e.g., Raghavan & Jain, 2016; Tsiligianni, Rodriguez, Lisspers, LeeTan, & Infantino, 2017). This is partially because of increased smoking in women (and greater lung damage due to smoking) as well as other factors such as sex hormones, occupational exposures, and comorbidities (Kamil, Pinzon, & Foreman, 2013; Raghavan & Jain, 2016). At the same degree of disease severity, women with COPD demonstrate greater disease burden (Global Initiative for Chronic Obstructive Lung Disease [GOLD], 2018), evidenced by greater physical impairment, dyspnea, emotional difficulties, and mortality (e.g., Cadeddu, Capizzi, Colombo, Nica, & De Belvis, 2016; Jenkins et al., 2017). Women are also often misdiagnosed, or their diagnosis is delayed (Cadeddu et al., 2016; Tsiligianni et al., 2017).

Asthma occurs more frequently in boys than in girls, but the sex difference reverses at puberty, so that asthma is more prevalent in adult women than men (e.g., Kynyk, Mastronarde, & McCallister, 2011; Zein & Erzurum, 2015). This is thought to be at least partially due to sex hormones that impact lung growth and development, but there are other confounding factors, such as obesity and environmental exposures (e.g., Kamil et al., 2013; Zein & Erzurum, 2015). Women also have more severe symptoms, including more dyspnea, depression, anxiety, physical limitations, and health care utilization, as well as decreased quality of life (Kynyk, Mastronarde, & McCallister, 2011; Zein & Erzurum, 2015).

Few studies have been done on sex differences in less prevalent chronic lung diseases, although sarcoidosis appears to occur more frequently in women (Gerke, Judson, Cozier, Culver, & Koth, 2017), and sleep apnea occurs more frequently in men (e.g., Snyder & Cunningham, 2018). There is no sex difference in the prevalence of cystic fibrosis (CF), but women have more severe disease, worse outcomes, and increased mortality (Raghavan & Jain, 2016).

Race and Ethnicity

Most studies of racial differences in chronic respiratory disease have been completed with asthma patients. An increased prevalence of asthma in African Americans has been documented repeatedly, as well as increased health care utilization, decreased asthma control, increased exacerbations and hospitalizations, and increased mortality (e.g., Canino, McQuaid, & Rand,

2009; Gold et al., 2013; McQuaid, 2018; Venkat et al., 2015). Apter et al. (2003) reported decreased adherence in African Americans with asthma, and others have noted low socioeconomic status and poor education as factors that interfere with adherence in this population (e.g., Canino et al., 2009; Gold et al., 2013; McQuaid, 2018). Furthermore, some researchers have reported on disparities in the treatment of asthma in African American patients. Specifically, African Americans with asthma are often provided treatment similar to other groups, even though they present with greater disease severity, which should make them *more* likely to be prescribed inhaled corticosteroids and to receive a referral to a specialist (Trent, Hasegawa, Ramratnam, Bittner, & Camargo, 2017; Venkat et al., 2015).

Cazzola, Calzetta, Matera, Hanania, and Rogliani (2018) provided an excellent review of the role of race and ethnicity in asthma treatment. They noted that ethnicity goes beyond the physical characteristics of race and includes additional cultural and social components. They reported that African American and Hispanic/Latinos are less responsive to asthma medications; this may be the result of genetic and environmental factors, as well as of factors associated with disease development. Worse outcomes in these minorities can be due to socioeconomic variables, differences in environmental exposures, decreased adherence, and decreased access to health care. Although a genetic component cannot be changed, many of these other variables can be addressed to improve asthma outcomes in minorities.

COPD is less prevalent in Blacks than in Whites, although it develops earlier in the African American population, and after less smoking (Foreman et al., 2011; Kamil et al., 2013). Furthermore, Blacks with COPD demonstrate more frequent exacerbations and poorer quality of life (Kamil et al., 2013). They are also less likely to be given advice to quit smoking (Kirkpatrick & Dransfield, 2009).

Sarcoidosis occurs most frequently in African American and northern European Whites. In the African American group, however, it presents at a younger age and results in more severe disease and increased mortality (Gerke, Judson, Cozier, Culver, & Koth, 2017).

Age

Most of the chronic respiratory diseases discussed here begin in middle age and become worse as people grow older. COPD, pulmonary fibrosis, pulmonary hypertension, and obstructive sleep apnea (OSA) tend to follow this pattern. However, sarcoidosis occurs most frequently in people ages 20 to 45 years, and it is less frequent in children and older patients (Short &

Ghio, 2016). Asthma occurs frequently in children but can begin anytime throughout the lifespan. CF is present at birth and tends to shorten the lifespan significantly, although many patients with CF now live into middle age.

Tobacco Smoking

Tobacco smoking is, by far, the most common contributing factor to the development of chronic respiratory disease, implicated in 80% to 90% of COPD cases (Wagena, Huibers, & van Schayck, 2001). It also plays a role in the development or exacerbation of asthma (U.S. Department of Health & Human Services, 2014), tuberculosis (Jeyashree, Kathirvel, Shewade, Kaur, & Goel, 2016), and IPF (Weinberger et al., 2019). Smoking cessation is the only treatment that can slow the progression of chronic lung disease (Jiménez-Ruiz et al., 2015). Because of the significance of smoking in the development of respiratory diseases, Chapter 8 is devoted to this topic exclusively and also includes details on interventions for smoking cessation.

Alcohol Use and Abuse

About 70% of adults in the United States drink alcohol (Substance Abuse and Mental Health Services Administration, 2019b), which can create problems in lung functioning (see Boé, Vandivier, Burnham, & Moss, 2009, for specific physiological mechanisms). Alcohol use or abuse can cause inflammation that can increase the likelihood of developing an infection. Several studies of alcohol *abuse* have demonstrated an increased risk of the development of acute respiratory diseases, such as acute respiratory distress syndrome and pneumonia; alcohol abuse in these patients was also associated with longer ICU stays, delayed recovery, increased duration of mechanical ventilation, and increased mortality (Boé et al., 2009).

The effects of alcohol use have been studied only minimally in chronic lung disease, so much information is yet unknown. However, alcohol can relax muscles and is associated with the development or worsening of OSA (e.g., Kolla et al., 2018; Taveira et al., 2018). In a challenge with asthma patients, alcohol resulted in histamine release, causing bronchoconstriction in about half of the subjects, suggesting that alcohol use could result in asthma exacerbations (Matsuse, 2016).

Alcohol can also alter the effects of medications used to manage lung disease. Specifically, the effectiveness of glucocorticoids and antibiotics can be decreased in the context of alcohol, while the effects of others (e.g., pain medications) may be increased (Leader, 2019). In addition, recovery after surgery can be affected by alcohol use. One study demonstrated that lung transplant patients who used alcohol minimally spent more time on a ventilator, in the ICU, and in the hospital overall than those who did not (Lowery, Yong, Cohen, Joyce, & Kovacs, 2018). Chronic respiratory patients would do well to avoid drinking alcohol completely, or use it only minimally, and should be referred to their doctor to get information on the specific impacts it could have, given their particular medical situation.

Health Literacy

Defined as "the degree to which individuals have the capacity to obtain, process, and understand basic health information and services needed to make appropriate health decisions" (U.S. Department of Health and Human Services, Office of Disease Prevention and Health Promotion, 2010, p. iii), *poor health literacy* is found in as many as 90 million Americans (Institute of Medicine, 2004). It affects a patient's management of their disease and also clinical outcomes. In the context of chronic respiratory disease, asthma patients with poor health literacy demonstrate decreased adherence, misconceptions about asthma, and poor inhaler technique (Federman et al., 2014; Soones et al., 2017). COPD patients with poor health literacy demonstrate decreased adherence, greater disease severity, greater helplessness, decreased respiratory quality of life, increased comorbidities, decreased knowledge about the disease, a greater likelihood of anxiety and depression, and increased hospital and emergency department visits (O'Conor et al., 2019; Omachi, Sarkar, Yelin, Blanc, & Katz, 2013; Puente-Maestu et al., 2016). Health literacy can be easily measured by the mental health practitioner (see Chapter 4) and can then be addressed with additional education.

GENETICS

CF "is one of the most widespread autosomal recessive diseases in the world" (Priestley et al., 2017, p. 160), caused by a genetic mutation. The CF mutation is a protein that affects the balance of sodium and water in cells, creating the mucous secretions that cause problems within the lungs (and other organs). Individuals can be carriers of the CF gene, and a child whose parents are both carriers will have a 25% chance of being born with the disease (World Health Organization, 2015).

Alpha$_1$ antitrypsin deficiency, a deficiency of a blood protein, is the cause of COPD in some patients. Especially if an individual smokes, this deficiency is associated with the early development of COPD (Weinberger et al., 2019). It is not yet clear how genetic factors may play a role in most cases of COPD.

Children with asthma may have a family history of allergies or asthma, although no specific genetic pattern has been delineated (Weinberger et al., 2019). A small percentage of cases of pulmonary hypertension are inherited, with a genetic mutation that impacts smooth muscle cell growth (although patients without a family history of the disease demonstrate the same mutation; Weinberger et al., 2019). Other chronic pulmonary diseases, such as sarcoidosis and OSA, seem to have no genetic component that contributes to their development or course.

CONCLUSION

Some of the factors that affect the development and course of chronic respiratory disease cannot be changed, such as gender, ethnicity, and genetics. For others, however, behavioral changes can have a large impact, for example, for a patient who quits smoking or who works in an environment that minimizes occupational exposures. Health literacy, on the other hand, can be addressed through education and clear communication.

PART II PSYCHOLOGICAL INTERVENTION

4 PSYCHOLOGICAL EVALUATION OF PULMONARY PATIENTS

The goals for the psychological evaluation of the pulmonary patient are to assess the patient's psychological and cognitive status, make recommendations, and provide feedback to the patient and the referral source. Although the main purpose is to evaluate the patient, brief intervention may also be provided during the interview. The specific format of the evaluation will depend on a variety of factors, including whether the evaluation is completed on an inpatient or an outpatient basis. The main focus in this book is on outpatient evaluations.

REFERRALS

Pulmonary patients are typically referred to the psychologist by a pulmonologist or a primary care physician who is looking for help in managing psychological problems that may be complicating the medical treatment. Alternatively, patients may self-refer. The most common referral questions from physicians involve depression, anxiety, nonadherence, and cognitive changes. Patients are most likely to self-refer with concerns about mood, stress, and coping, although they may not use those terms.

http://dx.doi.org/10.1037/0000189-005

Depression is a common referral question. Symptoms of depression may reflect a new problem that is due to difficulty adjusting to physical limitations associated with the lung disease or due to a premorbid depression that existed prior to a diagnosis of pulmonary disease. Similarly, patients may demonstrate premorbid anxiety or new onset anxiety symptoms secondary to pulmonary symptoms (e.g., breathlessness) or as a side effect of a medical treatment (e.g., theophylline, a bronchodilator, can cause restlessness and increased heart rate). Patients may be nonadherent to medications, pulmonary rehabilitation, or other treatments, either intentionally or otherwise. Finally, patients may demonstrate cognitive changes that may be temporary (due to decreased oxygen) or permanent (due to a dementia that is unrelated to the pulmonary disease).

Exhibit 4.1 lists some specific referral questions and issues for the psychologist to consider when evaluating the patient. Note the overlap between the psychological and medical symptoms (e.g., is shortness of breath [SOB] due to anxiety or chronic obstructive pulmonary disease [COPD]?). The psychologist will need to sort out the etiology of the symptoms to ascertain the correct diagnosis. More details on the overlap between psychological and respiratory symptoms can be found in the chapters on anxiety and depression.

EXHIBIT 4.1. Common Referral Questions for Pulmonary Patients

Referral	Issues to consider/assess
Patient with low energy, seems depressed	Clinical depression or depressed mood; low energy due to shortness of breath (SOB) or decreased interest or both?
Patient started on oxygen, seems depressed	Difficulty adjusting? Hypoxic?
Patient argumentative with family	Cognitive changes? How is social support? Patient with new limitations and frustration?
Patient hospitalized after skipping meds	Does patient understand the regimen? Forgetful? Intentionally not taking them?
Patient with SOB but no asthma attack	What are triggers for SOB? Anxiety?
Patient giving up on chronic obstructive pulmonary disease treatment	Does patient need help managing a complicated regimen? Depression? Suicidal ideation?
Patient not doing chest physiotherapy	Adjustment problems? Needs help with it? Understands the importance of this?

MEDICAL RECORD REVIEW

When it is available, the psychologist should review the patient's medical record. The purpose of this review is to gain an understanding of the medical issues that the patient is dealing with as well as any history of psychological symptoms. The clinician will want to know the patient's pulmonary diagnosis as well as the specific symptoms that the patient experiences. Previous notes from any mental health professionals can provide important information about premorbid psychological problems and past treatments. Medications can be reviewed, with special attention to psychotropic and other drugs that can result in psychological symptoms. In the medical record review, the mental health provider might learn, for instance, that a patient has been newly diagnosed with asthma, has been taking an anxiolytic for several years, and has been to the emergency room several times with what appeared to be panic attacks; such information provides preliminary hypotheses about the patient's problems and can help to guide the interview with the patient.

If the patient is seen outside of a medical center, there may be no medical record to review. At times, and with the patient's permission, the medical records can be requested, or the psychologist may consult directly with the referring physician to get information on the medical history and referral concerns. If the patient is self-referred, much of the history can be obtained from the patient, and the records request or consultation with the physician may happen after the interview.

PATIENT INTERVIEW

Exhibit 4.2 lists specific information to be obtained in the initial interview with the patient. Note that this is largely a generic evaluation but with a focus on the respiratory issues and their impacts on the patient. If the patient is self-referred, it is best to start with the patient's presenting problem; otherwise, the order of the interview items is less relevant.

Medical History

The clinician will want to hear from the patient about the pulmonary disease in detail, even if she has a good understanding of it from the medical record review. The goals here are to determine the specific symptoms and their impact on the patient's life and to assess his understanding of the disease,

EXHIBIT 4.2. Interview for Respiratory Patients

Medical history and current issues:

    Respiratory disease: diagnosis, symptoms, severity, frequency, duration, impacts (physical and psychological)

    Treatments for pulmonary disease—past and current

    Other medical problems

    Current medications

Adherence to current regimen:

    Barriers to adherence

    Past nonadherence

Social situation:

    Marital status/kids/living situation

    Education

    Employment

    Social support

Substance use:

    Current use/history of problems/past treatment

    Tobacco

    Alcohol

    Drugs

Psychiatric history and current treatment:

    Previous psychiatric treatment—inpatient and outpatient

    Psychotropic medications

    Family psychiatric history

    Suicide attempts, self-harm

    Current psychological/psychiatric treatment

Current psychological status:

    Mood/depression

    Sleep/appetite

    Guilt/worthlessness

    Interest

    Energy

    Hopelessness/helplessness

    Suicidal ideation

    Irritability

    Anxiety

    Worry

    Panic

    Manic symptoms

    Paranoia

    Hallucinations

EXHIBIT 4.2. Interview for Respiratory Patients (*Continued*)

Mental status:
  Subjective cognitive assessment
  Orientation
  Registration
  Attention/calculation
  Long-term memory
  Abstract thinking
  Judgment
  Short-term memory
  Behavioral observations
  Health literacy

Coping:
  Typical coping strategies and effectiveness
  Coping with pulmonary disease and symptoms

Special topics:
  Lung transplantation
  Decisional capacity

Note. Adapted from *Health Psychology Consultation in the Inpatient Medical Setting* (pp. 67–68), by S. M. Labott, 2019, Washington, DC: American Psychological Association. Copyright 2019 by the American Psychological Association.

its implications, and treatment recommendations. A patient's description of the disease, symptoms, and impact often provides important information about the patient's management of the disease as well as emotional coping.

The mental health clinician will also want to obtain information on any other medical issues with which the patient is currently dealing, as these can have significant effects on the patient's life and/or disease process. For example, older people with COPD are likely to have additional chronic medical problems, such as lung cancer, cardiovascular disease, osteoporosis, or gastroesophageal reflux disease (Global Initiative for Chronic Obstructive Lung Disease, 2018). Comorbidities such as these, in combination with the pulmonary disease, can increase the burden on the patient, which may be reflected in poor quality of life, decreased adherence to the medical regimen, or psychological symptoms. Even temporary conditions can play a role. A patient with cystic fibrosis (CF), for example, who is younger and may not have other chronic medical conditions, may have difficulty complying with chest physiotherapy if he is suffering from a recent back injury.

Adherence

Adherence is a significant problem in all medical treatment, especially in patients with chronic respiratory diseases. Patients should be asked about their success at following each aspect of the regimen (e.g., exercise, medication) and about any barriers to adherence that they experience. Nonadherence can take several forms, such as failure to adopt the treatment regimen, stopping treatment too soon, taking too much or too little of a medication, inconsistent adherence, or problems with the timing of medications (Dunbar-Jacob, Schlenk, & McCall, 2012).

The factor that accounts for most nonadherence problems is the complexity of the treatment regimen. Complex regimens occur often in diseases such as COPD, in which a patient must take oral medications, use inhalers, and attend pulmonary rehabilitation. Nonadherence can occur because patients do not understand the regimen, so they make mistakes in following it, or because they do not believe that following the regimen will improve their health. They may skip medications because they cannot pay for them or because they cannot reach their doctor to ask a question. Chapter 5 discusses adherence in more detail and includes a case study.

Social Situation

The topics of family, education, and employment should be discussed. For pulmonary patients, these topics will provide context. This will yield information about social stressors apart from the disease and also important data on daily activities that may be limited by the respiratory problem.

Social support can influence how patients manage their disease. People with physical limitations may need others to help around the house or take them to medical appointments (*instrumental support*), and most patients will benefit from supportive others who help keep them positive and motivated (*emotional support*).

Substance Use

Because smoking is strongly associated with several pulmonary diseases, current and past tobacco use need to be assessed, including what the person has smoked, how much daily, and over what time period. Past quit efforts, as well as successes and failures associated with them, should also be discussed. Patients may experience guilt at their failures and feel helpless to make changes currently. Current and past alcohol and drug use should also be assessed. Any past treatments for alcohol or drug abuse are also relevant.

Psychiatric History and Current Treatment

As with any new patient, past psychological and psychiatric treatments should be discussed. Information on psychotropic medications taken, and if they have provided relief or not, should be determined. Any past psychological therapy should be asked about, including what the patient felt worked in the treatment and what did not. Psychiatric inpatient admissions should be discussed, including when they happened and for what reasons. Suicide attempts, other self-harm, and family history of psychiatric problems should also be determined. Current treatments will also need to be discussed. Current medications and psychotherapy will need to be delineated as well as the patient's feelings about them.

Current Psychological Status

Exhibit 4.2 contains a list of psychological symptoms that patients may experience; the psychologist will want to determine which are currently experienced by the patient as well as their severity and impact on the patient's day-to-day functioning. This includes symptoms of anxiety, depression, and psychosis. The role (if any) of respiratory symptoms in the production of these psychological symptoms will need to be determined. That is, a patient may experience depressed mood only when he has to tell his granddaughter that he cannot walk her to the park and push her on the swing, or he experiences anxiety when he is exerting himself climbing stairs and cannot breathe. In other cases, patients have experienced the anxiety or depression symptoms throughout their lives (prior to the development of respiratory disease), but the respiratory disease now exacerbates the preexisting psychological symptoms.

Mental Status

A formal mental status examination should be performed at all new evaluations with pulmonary patients. Cognitive impairment has been demonstrated in patients with chronic pulmonary disease (Andrianopoulos, Gloeckl, Vogiatzis, & Kenn, 2017; Torres-Sánchez et al., 2015). It is often caused by poor oxygenation, and elderly patients are more susceptible to it than younger patients. There are several commonly used measures that are quickly administered and provide good screening for cognitive problems. The Mini-Mental State Exam (MMSE; Folstein, Folstein, & McHugh, 1975) takes only a few minutes to administer and provides data on basic cognitive tasks, such as orientation, short- and long-term memory, attention, and language.

The Modified Mini-Mental State Examination (Teng & Chui, 1987) is based on the MMSE but includes additional items and assesses additional domains (e.g., similarities). Norms are available for both (e.g., Boustani et al., 2003; Bravo & Hébert, 1997). These screeners can provide an estimate of a patient's cognitive functioning and can also be used to track changes in cognition over time.

Patients should be asked questions about their subjective cognitive functioning, for example:

- Do you have concerns about your memory?
- Do you ever feel confused?
- Do you ever forget something important?
- Do you notice any changes in your thinking recently, or have others noticed?

Patients can also be asked to respond to additional items to assess a specific ability in more detail or to assess other cognitive abilities (see Strub & Black, 2000, for more mental status screening tasks). Finally, behavioral observations can provide data on fatigue, breathlessness, affect, and self-care.

Health literacy can have dramatic impacts on a patient's ability to understand and manage chronic respiratory diseases; it may result in difficulty understanding the disease and the regimen as well as problems communicating clearly with providers. Health literacy is easily assessed, and several measures are available to do so. Using the Rapid Estimate of Adult Literacy in Medicine—Short Form (Arozullah et al., 2007), the clinician asks patients to read seven medical words out loud. This takes only a few minutes; a higher number of words pronounced correctly reflects a higher reading level and greater health literacy. A similar measure, the Short Assessment of Health Literacy for Spanish Adults (S. D. Lee, Bender, Ruiz, & Cho, 2006) is available for patients who speak Spanish.

Coping

The clinician will want to assess how patients cope with stressors or problems in their lives. It is helpful to know if patients face problems or if they avoid or deny them. Do they take measures to try to solve problems, do they seek additional information to help them, or do they seek social support to help them manage?

Coping specifically with the respiratory symptoms and disease should also be discussed. Patients may have new physical or cognitive limitations, which may affect their work or their role in the family. They may experience emotional distress and psychological symptoms that are new to them. What coping strategies has the patient used that have helped them to manage the disease? What have they tried that has not worked? Chapter 5 contains details on enabling coping for those patients who need it, and Exhibit 5.2 is a list of coping strategies that patients may use.

Special Topics

For some evaluations, there may be additional topics to be discussed, or certain topics for which more detail is needed. In a lung transplant evaluation, not only will general social support need to be assessed, but the patient will need a supportive person who will commit to significant instrumental and emotional support throughout the process, because this is inevitably a requirement for transplantation. It will also need to be determined that the patient has the ability and willingness to follow a complex treatment regimen. Some emotional issues may need to be assessed in more detail (e.g., concerns about the process, guilt). Finally, the psychologist should remember that people being evaluated for transplant are motivated to present themselves in the best light possible so that they are approved for the transplant; this will need to be managed during the evaluation so that conclusions are as accurate as possible.

Another specialized evaluation may be required for a patient whose decisional capacity is in question (see also Chapter 10). Generally, the concern is if the patient is able to make decisions about specific medical treatments. Decisional capacity requires that the person is able to communicate his or her wishes about the proposed treatment, understands the relevant information and the consequences of the decision, and can rationally manipulate information (e.g., Appelbaum & Grisso, 1988; Leo, 1999; Searight, 1992). Specific questions to assess these domains as well as information on standardized measures that are available to help with a decisional capacity assessment can be found in Labott (2019).

PSYCHOLOGICAL TESTING

For patients who raise concerns about cognitive functioning, neuropsychological testing is appropriate. Because chronic pulmonary patients are often required to follow a complex medical regimen, providers need to have confidence that they are cognitively able to manage it. If a patient does present with cognitive impairments, plans can be developed to help her to manage specific tasks or to ensure that she remains safe.

Brief interview or self-report measures can also be administered to patients to provide additional information on various aspects of their functioning, such as psychological symptoms, quality of life, and their experience and reactions to symptoms of lung disease. These measures can also be used to monitor a patient's progress over time. Exhibit 4.3 lists some common measures that may be useful. These are most helpful if the psychologist selects the measure(s) most relevant for a specific patient and his situation.

EXHIBIT 4.3. Brief Assessment Measures for Pulmonary Patients

General functioning:

Patient Health Questionnaire (PHQ; Spitzer, Kroenke, & Williams, 1999; PHQ-9, Kroenke, Spitzer, & Williams, 2001): Measure depression (PHQ, PHQ-9) and anxiety (PHQ)

Short Form Health Survey (SF-36; Ware & Sherbourne, 1992): Measures limitations due to medical problems, mental health, overall perspective on current health

Millon Behavioral Medicine Diagnostic (Millon, Antoni, Millon, Minor, & Grossman, 2001): Measures psychosocial factors that may impact the patient's medical treatment

Beck Depression Inventory–II (Beck, Steer, & Brown, 1996): A brief and commonly used measure of symptoms of depression

Measures specific to respiratory illness:

Quality of life

   Cystic Fibrosis Questionnaire (Quittner, Buu, Messer, Modi, & Watrous, 2005): Measures effects of cystic fibrosis on health and daily life

   Cough Quality of Life Questionnaire (French, Irwin, Fletcher, & Adams, 2002): Measures how cough impacts the individual's life and reactions to it

   Asthma Quality of Life Questionnaire (Juniper et al., 1992): Patients are interviewed about activities that cause them most difficulty due to asthma

   Assessment of Burden of COPD (ABC) Scale (Slok et al., 2016): Assesses symptoms, physical limitations, and emotional reactions due to chronic obstructive pulmonary disease symptoms

   Chronic Respiratory Questionnaire (Guyatt, Berman, Townsend, Pugsley, & Chambers, 1987): This interview examines the major activities in which the patient experiences dyspnea and emotional reactions

Breathlessness

   UCSD Shortness-of-Breath Questionnaire (Eakin, Resnikoff, Prewitt, Ries, & Kaplan, 1998): Assesses shortness of breath when engaging in 21 physical activities, with three items about limitations

   Shortness of Breath With Daily Activities (Watkins et al., 2013): Patients rate their shortness of breath for 13 physical activities

   Breathlessness Beliefs Questionnaire (De Peuter et al., 2011): 17 items measure anxiety associated with dyspnea

   Dyspnoea-12 Questionnaire (Yorke, Moosavi, Shuldham, & Jones, 2010): A 12-item questionnaire that assesses general shortness of breath and emotional reactions

COLLATERAL INFORMATION

There are a variety of situations in which it will be necessary to contact a family member (with the patient's permission) to get additional information; anyone close to the patient who spends significant time with the patient can be interviewed if the family is unavailable or unaware of the patient's recent behavior. This contact might be warranted in cases in which a patient evidences cognitive changes and does not remember certain information. At other times, patients recall the information but are unable to articulate it (e.g., due to difficulty breathing or problems communicating if on a ventilator). Other patients are less than truthful about their history, often when reporting drug or alcohol abuse. In these cases, family or friends can provide accurate information.

Because the patient's significant others are usually not used to carefully observing and reporting on the patient's behavior, it will be important for the clinician to ask clear (and jargon-free) questions. Sample questions include the following: Have you noticed any changes in the patient's thinking? Any confusion? Is he behaving any differently with other people? Do you know how much and how often she drinks alcohol?

FEEDBACK

At the conclusion of the interview, it will be important to provide feedback to the patient. This can take the form of a brief summary of the information the patient has provided, followed by the clinician's understanding of the relevant psychological issues and recommendations for how to address them. This should be done in clear language that the patient can easily understand, and the patient's experiences should be normalized, rather than labeled as *mental illness*. After all of the information obtained during the evaluation is integrated, including testing data and collateral information, a formal report should be provided to the referral source (discussed more thoroughly in Chapter 11). Case 4.1 presents an evaluation of a young man with CF.

A SPECIAL POPULATION: PEOPLE WITH MEDICALLY UNEXPLAINED RESPIRATORY SYMPTOMS

The psychologist may receive a referral on a patient who is presenting to the pulmonary clinic with medically unexplained respiratory symptoms. That is, after a thorough medical workup has been completed, there is no cause found to account for the symptoms. The most common unexplained respiratory symptoms are cough (referred to as *psychogenic cough, habit cough,*

CASE 4.1
CYSTIC FIBROSIS EVALUATION

Patient (pt) is a 24-year-old Caucasian man who lives with his parents. He is not currently employed or attending school.

Pt was diagnosed with CF as a baby. Throughout his life, he has had recurrent lung infections, many of which have resulted in hospitalizations. Pt missed many days in grammar school due to illness but managed to not be held back. In high school, he reports not taking care of himself, was sick more often, missed a lot of school, and eventually dropped out. Neither the pt nor his parents were concerned about this at the time because none of them expected him to live into his 20s. In high school he dated, but he didn't take relationships seriously because he didn't think he would be alive long enough to have a long-term relationship or a family.

Pt reports no medical problems besides CF. He also reports that he is currently adherent to his medications, participates in chest physiotherapy, and follows the nutritional guidelines he has been given. He noted this is a bit of a burden, but he now understands the importance of following the treatment regimen. Pt denied that CF symptoms have a significant impact on his daily activities; he completed the Cystic Fibrosis Questionnaire, which confirmed that symptoms only minimally impact his functioning. Results also indicated, however, that his quality of life is poor, especially in terms of social and role limitations.

Pt reports drinking beer "occasionally" and denies drinking daily or to excess. He denies use of tobacco or drugs and reports no history of problems with any substances.

Pt reports seeing a counselor briefly in high school; otherwise, no formal psych treatment. He thinks he is depressed currently. He reports depressed mood most of the time, poor sleep, poor social support (none except for parents), and feelings of giving up. He denies suicidal ideation, significant anxiety, manic, or psychotic symptoms. He does report worry about his future. He also reports feeling bored because he doesn't have much to do.

Pt denies subjective cognitive problems. On mental status exam he was alert and oriented × 3. Registration, attention, short- and long-term memory are all intact. Judgment was OK on assessment. Speech normal in rate and rhythm; mood appears slightly depressed. Pt appears younger than his stated age.

Conclusions:

Pt with CF, struggling to cope with its implications. Because he did not think he would live into his 20s, he has not worked to complete his education, to gain employment, or to develop important relationships. He is socially isolated, with depressed mood. His compliance with CF treatment is currently good.

CASE 4.1
CYSTIC FIBROSIS EVALUATION (*Continued*)

Discussed with pt the following recommendations:

1. Vocational testing or counseling to help him seek appropriate employment or volunteer work
2. CF support group to decrease isolation and increase social support
3. Outpatient behavioral medicine treatment to help him develop realistic expectations for his future, to increase activity generally, and to improve mood and sleep

or *unexplained cough*), sneezing (*paroxysmal sneezing*), wheezing and dyspnea (*paradoxical vocal cord dysfunction; PVCD*), or *functional aphonia* or *dysphonia* (loss of voice and difficulty in voice production, respectively). People with medically unexplained symptoms are often angry and feel that providers do not believe them, even though the symptoms are often quite obvious (e.g., continual coughing).

These are appropriate referrals for a psychologist, but it is not the case that simply because there is no clear medical cause for the symptom, it must be psychiatric in nature. In the evaluation, the psychologist will want to work to build rapport and to specifically attend to the possibility of anxiety, somatoform, or factitious disorders. Even if psychological symptoms or disorders are present, there are several reasons why it should rarely be concluded that the respiratory symptoms are caused exclusively by psychological factors: (a) Many medically unexplained symptoms are subclinical initially and undetectable by current diagnostic tests, but in the future they might be diagnosed as respiratory illnesses; (b) we have no way to know definitively that the symptoms are caused *exclusively* by psychological and not medical factors (although it is common for psychological factors to play a role); (c) if the psychologist concludes the symptoms are the result of psychiatric factors, the pulmonologist will stop treating the patient, which will make it certain that a respiratory cause is never found; and (d) this finding labels the patient as a psychiatric case and confirms what others have likely already told her (i.e., "it is all in your head"). In an evaluation of this type the psychologist can generally identify factors that exacerbate or maintain the symptom and can then intervene to help the patient with behavioral and cognitive strategies to manage the symptom (without labeling the symptom as a *psychological disorder*). Speech therapy is also useful in the treatment of PVCD and functional voice disorders. A recommendation that the physician continue to follow the patient is usually also warranted.

5 ADJUSTMENT

The term *adjustment* can be used to refer to the process through which a patient adapts to lung disease, or it can be used to refer to the end state of successful adaptation. In this chapter, the focus is not on adjustment *disorders*; rather, it is on the natural process that occurs when a patient is faced with new or changing medical issues. For pulmonary patients, adjustment involves dealing with physical changes and limitations and coming to terms emotionally with the symptoms and the disease.

ADJUSTMENT TO CHRONIC LUNG DISEASE

Hoyt and Stanton (2012) reviewed the literature on adjustment in chronic illness and reported that successful adjustment is conceptualized by researchers in several different ways: (a) the mastery of tasks associated with the illness, (b) a lack of psychopathology, (c) decreased negative or increased positive affect, (d) good functional status, and (e) positive quality of life. Exhibit 5.1 translates these conceptualizations into specific tasks associated with adjustment for pulmonary patients. Note that the best

http://dx.doi.org/10.1037/0000189-006
Psychological Treatment of Patients With Chronic Respiratory Disease, by S. M. Labott

EXHIBIT 5.1. Patient Tasks Associated With Successful Adjustment to Chronic Lung Disease

Understand the disease and related issues
  Typical disease course; the adjustment process
  Causes of exacerbations and triggers of symptoms
  Rationale for treatments, such as nebulizer, medications, rehabilitation

Adhere to medical recommendations
  Proper use of the treatments, for example, when to take medication, how to use inhaler
  Skills and ability to adhere to the treatment regimen

Cope successfully with symptoms, limitations, and emotional reactions
  Appropriate expectations
  Behaviors to compensate for limitations, for example, pacing activities
  Willingness to use aids to improve functioning

Develop feelings of control and self-efficacy

adjustment occurs when a patient understands the disease and its implications, adheres to the treatment regimen, is able to cope successfully, and feels able to manage the symptoms and disease. Clinically, patients may be evaluated with respect to their abilities on each of the dimensions in Exhibit 5.1, and then weaker areas can be addressed through treatment to improve the patients' adaptation and functioning (see the next section, Intervention).

Many pulmonary diseases are diagnosed when patients complain of dyspnea on exertion. Patients have become aware of new symptoms, such as shortness of breath, cough, or sputum production, and they begin to accommodate so that they can perform the activities they want to, although typically more slowly and with less exertion. As a progressive disease worsens, the physical limitations become more pronounced, and patients may need to use aids (e.g., cane, wheelchair) to help them function comfortably. Later, in the case of severe illness, people may need to give up some activities completely and use supplemental oxygen to breathe comfortably. At initial diagnosis and at times of significant change in a patient's medical situation, she may feel overwhelmed and experience a variety of emotions such as fear, anxiety, and sadness. As described later, education about the disease can help to decrease a patient's fears.

Fear is a common response when people feel short of breath; note these comments from patients:

> It's the worst feeling in the world . . . the worst way to die . . . it's like smothering to death . . . and you think life is coming to an end, everything is over . . .

it's the scariest situation . . . to lose control of your breathing . . . you wonder if you'll make it or not. (DeVito, 1990, p. 188)

When people become afraid, their breathing becomes worse, which then results in more fear, creating a cycle (Willgoss, Yohannes, Goldbart, & Fatoye, 2012). People may become fearful of experiencing dyspnea and may limit their activity more than is medically necessary to avoid these unpleasant feelings.

Patients may also experience anxiety about new medical procedures. They may have fears about what their future will hold, especially as they often have little knowledge initially of what a diagnosis of pulmonary disease will mean to them. They may also grieve about losses they are currently or may be facing in the future, such as the inability to play with grandchildren, continue their employment, or complete their chores around the house. They may lose valuable social contacts if they are unable to participate in sports or shop with friends. Many patients experience guilt if they believe they have brought this disease on themselves (e.g., by smoking).

Patients may deny the fact that they have a chronic lung disease and may refuse to change their behavior, take medication, or engage in any other treatment. Some patients resist initially but, over time, realize that following the medical regimen will help them be more comfortable and may increase their lifespan. Those who continue to resist, however, are likely to experience negative medical outcomes, such as increased shortness of breath and more frequent hospital admissions.

Even if patients accept their disease generally, they may be resistant to using physical aids, such as canes, walkers, and scooters. Many will refuse completely and may then struggle to ambulate or may fall and injure themselves. The resistance may be due to self-consciousness that others will negatively evaluate them because of the aid, or to denial that there is a physical issue that they need to address.

Because adjustment is a process, as the medical issues change, the patient will need to readjust to the new situation. For example, one patient was diagnosed with mild chronic obstructive pulmonary disease (COPD) at 40 years old and learned to make a few changes to her lifestyle to accommodate her new limitations (e.g., no strenuous physical activity). For many years she functioned well physically and emotionally. By age 55, the disease had significantly worsened, and she needed to make additional changes to adjust to the new scenario (e.g., pace all physical activity, use supplemental oxygen when sleeping).

INTERVENTION

Interventions to facilitate adjustment in patients with chronic lung disease are designed to help patients master the skills listed in Exhibit 5.1. These generally involve psychoeducation, coping skills training, and strategies to manage symptoms, emotions, and adherence.

Psychoeducation

Patients will initially need basic information on pulmonary physiology, the typical disease course, the recommended treatments, and how to administer them properly. Patients should learn about the disease generally as well as seek information relative to their specific medical situation. Much of this initial education will be done by the patient's medical team; information can then be reviewed and processed by the patient with the help of the psychologist.

It will be important for patients to become aware of specific triggers of their symptoms (e.g., pollutants) and those factors that decrease their specific symptoms (e.g., rest, pursed-lip breathing). A discussion about their experiences with their symptoms can help to delineate these patterns; some patients will not be aware of these patterns and will learn through trial and error.

Patients will need specific information on the medical treatments that their doctor has prescribed, including the rationale for all recommendations. They will need clear instructions regarding the use of all prescriptions, such as proper dosing and when to take a medication. If the medical recommendations include the use of new equipment, such as inhalers, nebulizers, supplemental oxygen, or chest physiotherapy devices, patients will need education as well as specific hands-on training in the use of these devices. Any barriers to adherence should also be discussed so that plans can be made to avoid interference with the patient's medical treatment.

Education will also be necessary for patients who need to use aids to help them ambulate. Specifically, patients need to understand that the goals are to improve their functioning and quality of life and to keep them safe. They will also need training to enable them to use these aids properly. When people understand that using the walker, cane, or other aids will allow them to participate in activities they enjoy, they are more likely to comply.

Patients can also benefit from education about the adjustment process itself. Many people feel overwhelmed when they realize they have a chronic illness that may change their lives, and they may feel unequipped to deal with it. Education about the normal adjustment process can lessen the feeling of being overwhelmed and make patients better able to cope with the situation. Specifically, patients can be told that adjustment is a process, that it will take time and effort to feel competent at handling it, and that they will need to continue to work on their strategies to manage over time. They can be encouraged to strive to be a resilient person who actively copes with these new challenges, rather than seeing themselves as a sick person with no agency and no power. They should be aware that emotional reactions, such as sadness or anxiety, are common, but that these can also be successfully managed. Most important, patients should be made aware that adjustment is a normal process (i.e., not a pathology) and that they will be able to learn to adapt successfully and to have a reasonable quality of life.

Promoting Adherence

Nonadherence is a significant problem in medical treatment generally, and it is worse in pulmonary disease than in other chronic diseases (e.g., DiMatteo, 2004b; Rolnick, Pawloski, Hedblom, Asche, & Bruzek, 2013). Nonadherence may involve under- or overuse of a medication, taking oral medications or using inhalers at the incorrect time, skipping exercise, continuing to smoke (Bourbeau & Bartlett, 2008), or misusing inhalers or supplemental oxygen. The nonadherence may be accidental or intentional (M. George, 2018).

Much of the research on adherence has been done with patients diagnosed with COPD. Many researchers have reported poor compliance with inhalers in COPD patients, with rates ranging from 33% to 53% (e.g., Horvat, Locatelli, Kos, & Janeûic, 2018; Humenberger et al., 2018). Similar low adherence rates are found for oral medications (54%; Cecere et al., 2012), combinations of oral and inhaled medications (29%–56%; Ingebrigtsen et al., 2015), and oxygen therapy (60%; Gauthier et al., 2019). Researchers have also noted differences in adherence rates for COPD versus asthma patients such that COPD patients are more adherent than asthma patients (e.g., Brandstetter et al., 2017; Plaza et al., 2016); this is likely a result of the episodic nature of asthma symptoms.

There is an abundance of evidence that adherence to the medical regimen in COPD is associated with positive impacts. Many studies have reported that adherence to the medication regimen is associated with decreases in hospital admissions (e.g., Choi, Chung, & Han, 2014; van Boven et al., 2014), health care utilization, and mortality (e.g., Cushen et al., 2018). Nonadherence has been associated with increased anxiety and depression (Choi et al., 2014), decreased quality of life (van Boven et al., 2014), and increased symptoms (Mesquita et al., 2018). Good reviews of adherence in pulmonary patients, including assessment, causes, impacts, and strategies to improve adherence, can be found in Bourbeau and Bartlett (2008); Duarte-de-Araújo, Teixeira, Hespanhol, and Correia-de-Sousa (2018); M. George (2018); and Global Initiative for Asthma (2018).

The *ABC model of adherence* postulates that adherence has three aspects: (a) initiation, (b) implementation, and (c) persistence (Vrijens et al., 2012). Many factors affect adherence, including those associated with the patient himself or herself, the treatment, the disease, and the patient's relationship with the medical provider. A person can demonstrate problems with adherence to any aspect of the medical regimen, and adherence to one aspect (e.g., taking oral medications properly) does not predict adherence to a different behavior (e.g., using supplemental oxygen; Dunbar-Jacob, Gemmell, & Schlenk, 2009).

If problems with adherence occur, the psychologist should review the patient's understanding of the regimen and its importance, delineate factors that cause the nonadherence, and then develop strategies to help the patient comply with the medical recommendations. Much nonadherence stems from a patient's not understanding the regimen. Therefore, it is critical that people are educated about the treatment recommendations and what exactly they will need to do to comply with them. Nonadherence can also be due to poor motivation, depression, or inadequate support. Patients may not have enough money to pay for their medications, may forget, or may actively decide not to take them. The most successful psychological intervention will target the specific cause of the nonadherence.

Patient Factors

Studies of patients with COPD have demonstrated an association between a patient's beliefs about the specific necessity of a medication and adherence, although there are inconsistent findings with asthma patients (Brandstetter et al., 2017; Fischer et al., 2018). Satisfaction with the medication (e.g., Chrystyn et al., 2014) and an understanding about the illness and treatment options (e.g., Choi et al., 2014) are also associated with adherence. COPD patients with better adherence are more likely to follow the disease management routine, rather than varying it on the basis of how they feel or to fit their lifestyle, and they tend to take action rather than put up with a problem (J. George, Kong, Thoman, & Stewart, 2005). People with poorer cognitive status are less adherent to proper inhaler technique (Turan, Turan, & Mirici, 2017), and those with caregivers are more adherent than those without (R. B. Trivedi, Bryson, Udris, & Au, 2012).

Practically, patients who deny the existence of the disease or the need to treat it are likely to demonstrate adherence problems. It is useful to engage these patients in a discussion of their thoughts and beliefs about the disease, as well as the implications of their behavior for the disease course. Although they may not like it, they can often see that taking their medication is in their best interest.

Those resisting specific aids (e.g., supplemental oxygen or a wheelchair) can be asked to consider their ability to function with and without the aid, and how this will affect their daily activities. Articulating the expected reaction of others can also be useful; patients are correct that others will notice and will likely react with initial concern, asking questions about their disease that the patient might like to avoid. Ways to manage that can be discussed as well as the likelihood that once the initial surprise dissipates, others often demonstrate relatively quick acceptance.

Treatment Regimen

The complexity of the medical regimen is known to be the main factor that affects adherence in medical patients generally (Ingersoll & Cohen, 2008). In chronic pulmonary disease treatment, complexity may result from the need to take oral medications, use inhalers, and attend pulmonary rehab at various times of the day or week. It may also be due to the dosing frequency of medications (Ágh, Inotai, & Mészáros, 2011; Sanduzzi et al., 2014), the use of complicated devices to deliver medications (Braido et al., 2016), or the mode of delivery (e.g., inhaler vs. patch; Charles et al., 2010). Complexity may be decreased by performing several tasks at the same time of day, but, given the nature of pulmonary disease, that is often not possible. In such situations, reminders can be set up, caregivers can be enlisted to keep patients on track, or more training and education can be initiated.

Patients are more likely to adhere to a regimen if their behavior has clear and immediate consequences, such as using an inhaler when having an asthma attack. This immediately decreases symptoms, thus reinforcing the use of the inhaler; taking a morning medication that seems to make no difference is a harder behavior to maintain (Sanduzzi et al., 2014). Patients may not adhere to a prescribed medication if they experience unpleasant side effects (Bourbeau & Bartlett, 2008); for example, bronchodilators and steroids are used in the treatment of lung diseases and are associated with anxiety symptoms. Finally, patients may not take medications properly if they are unable to afford them. Directing patients to programs that offer medications at a lower cost can often remedy this problem (social workers often have information on such programs).

Disease Characteristics

Characteristics of the specific disease also affect adherence. As noted previously, because of the episodic nature of asthma, it is associated with lower adherence rates than COPD (e.g., Brandstetter et al., 2017; Plaza et al., 2016). Disease severity has also been associated with adherence, such that patients with more severe disease are more adherent to the treatment regimen (Humenberger et al., 2018).

Relationship With the Provider

Adherence is better in COPD patients who report good communication (e.g., Rogliani, Ora, Puxeddu, Matera, & Cazzola, 2017) and trust in their medical provider (e.g., Duarte-de-Araújo et al., 2018). One review reported that a patient's personal connection to the pharmacist and pharmacy staff was the most important factor in adherence to asthma medications (Donner et al., 2018). Provider expertise (Cecere et al., 2012) and availability can also play a role. The psychologist can often work with the patient to communicate more clearly with the provider to improve the relationship to impact treatment adherence.

Case 5.1 presents a patient referred to psychology with a nonadherence problem. The psychological evaluation delineated several specific factors that accounted for the nonadherence. Several interventions were then undertaken to address these specific factors.

CASE 5.1

ADHERENCE

Background

Patient is a 72-year-old woman diagnosed with asthma, attending a routine appointment with her pulmonologist. Her symptoms have been well-controlled for many years, with an inhaled corticosteroid each morning and a short acting beta$_2$-agonist as a rescue inhaler for acute exacerbations. She is widowed and lives alone; she denies any problems managing at home alone. When the patient was questioned about her adherence to the medical regimen, she appeared sheepish but denied any problems. When her refills for her morning inhaler were checked, however, it was clear that she had not been using this as prescribed. Her nurse reviewed what the medication is for, how and when she should use it, and the importance of using it as scheduled. The patient agreed with all of this and seemed to understand. The psychologist was called to further evaluate the non-adherence and any contributing psychological issues.

CASE 5.1
ADHERENCE (*Continued*)
Psychological Evaluation

The patient had no history of psychological problems or treatments and no current significant psychological symptoms. On mental status exam, the patient demonstrated mild problems with both short- and long-term memory. She acknowledged that she sometimes doesn't remember if she has taken her medication or not. She seemed to be functioning safely at home generally, with some help from her daughter.

The patient was widowed about a year ago and is quite isolated. Patient reports financial problems since her husband's death, and she admitted that she is using her daily inhaler every two days, to save money. She understands that she should use it daily, and she acknowledges that she felt better when she was using it daily, although even when she can afford it she sometimes forgets to use it.

Treatment

1. The psychologist consulted with a social worker, who knew that the maker of the patient's drug had a program to help out with drug costs for patients who can't afford their medication. She agreed to enroll the patient into this program so that the patient would pay less for her inhaler.

2. The patient's daughter was contacted; she and her mother agreed that the daughter would organize the patient's oral medications and inhalers for her so that she could clearly tell them apart, and would also get an alarm to remind the patient to take all her meds at the proper times. The patient's daughter also agreed to monitor the patient's functioning at home more closely, so that she could take additional action if the patient began to have more problems.

3. The patient agreed to meet with the psychologist for a few visits, to discuss ways for her to be more active and connected socially.

Outcome

After 3 months, the patient returned to see her pulmonologist, accompanied by her daughter. She was feeling generally well, and she reported she was now able to afford her inhaler. Her daughter had set up a system to remind the patient to use her medications and inhaler as prescribed, and this was successful most of the time. The patient continued to live alone and was doing OK there, with her daughter's help. Patient had met with the psychologist twice and had developed plans to be more involved in her church and also to invite friends to her house to socialize. She had some minimal success with these plans so far. She reported some depressed mood on occasion, associated with the death of her husband. She planned to continue to see the psychologist monthly to work on these remaining issues.

Coping With Symptoms, Limitations, and Emotional Reactions

Lazarus and Folkman (1984) defined *coping* as "the constantly changing cognitive and behavioral efforts to manage specific external and/or internal demands that are appraised as taxing or exceeding the resources of the person" (p. 141). *Coping* refers to the strategies people use to manage stressors or to help them adapt. Patients have preferred strategies that they have used to cope with adversity throughout their lives; these strategies should be discussed and enhanced to the extent that they will help the patient to manage the lung disease. If patients do not have existing coping strategies sufficient to enable them to cope effectively, additional coping strategies can be learned.

Exhibit 5.2 contains a list of coping strategies and examples of applications for pulmonary patients. Consider the patient (above) who is fearful

EXHIBIT 5.2. Coping Strategies and Examples of Their Use With Pulmonary Patients

Planning/problem-solving	Making a schedule for new medications and pulmonary rehabilitation appointments
Active coping	Attend to symptoms; use medications and aids as recommended
Seeking instrumental or emotional support	Enlist help from friends for physically taxing chores; attend support group
Religious coping	Prayer and church attendance to increase feelings of support
Acceptance	Dealing with the reality of the situation
Positive reappraisal	Seeing the benefits of quitting smoking or engaging in appropriate exercise
Denial	Refusing to accept the diagnosis or make changes to manage the disease
Disengagement/distancing	Ignoring or removing oneself emotionally or physically from the situation
Wishful thinking	Unrealistic fantasizing about being disease free
Humor	Finding something funny about the situation; making light of it
Substance use; overeating	Overusing drugs, alcohol, or food to avoid addressing the problem
Taking responsibility	Realizing one needs to exert as much control as possible over the symptoms/disease
Distraction	Engaging in activities to avoid thinking about lung disease and its implications

Note. Adapted from *Health Psychology Consultation in the Inpatient Medical Setting* (p. 114), by S. M. Labott, 2019, Washington, DC: American Psychological Association. Copyright 2019 by the American Psychological Association.

when she becomes short of breath. This could be handled in several ways: Problem-solving strategies could help the patient develop plans to manage when she is short of breath: using an inhaler, sitting down to rest and relax, or using cognitive techniques that focus on calming herself rather than catastrophizing. She could also read or watch TV in an effort to distract herself from her fears.

Some of the strategies in Exhibit 5.2 are more adaptive than others. Studies of coping in COPD patients have reported that better quality of life and less emotional distress are associated with problem-solving (Andenaes, Kalfoss, & Wahl, 2006) and proactive coping (Tiemensma, Gaab, Voorhaar, Asijee, & Kaptein, 2016). Some strategies may serve a purpose temporarily but become less adaptive over time (e.g., denial), and others are not generally adaptive at all (e.g., disengagement, substance use).

Some respiratory patients may experience strong emotional reactions such as fear, anger, or sadness. Addressing these can be important as the clinician helps the patient come to terms with his situation. However, therapists should remain mindful of the underlying respiratory disease (and its severity) when working on intense emotional issues. These reactions can tax a patient's respiratory system and increase breathlessness; therefore, the experience and expression of strong emotions will need to be monitored and titrated for some respiratory patients, especially those with severe disease.

Developing Feelings of Control and Self-Efficacy

The literature on adjustment in respiratory patients acknowledges the importance of psychological factors, because pulmonary function alone does not account for a patient's quality of life or successful adjustment. This is consistent with Bandura's (1997) theory of the role of self-efficacy in chronic disease: A patient's functioning is more strongly related to self-efficacy than to physical impairments. Kohler, Fish, and Greene (2002) reported that the relationship between pulmonary symptoms and impairment in COPD patients is mediated by self-efficacy. Others have reported that self-efficacy in COPD patients is associated with improved quality of life, less depression and anxiety, and improved medication adherence (e.g., McCathie, Spence, & Tate, 2002; Popa-Velea & Purcarea, 2014).

Motivation and self-efficacy can be influenced using techniques of motivational interviewing (also discussed in Chapter 8). The point is to get patients to talk about change—this can be done by asking them to rate (a) how much they want to make a change and (b) how confident they are they could do it (Resnicow et al., 2002). The therapist and patient can then discuss the health behaviors that could improve the patient's life. Once the patient accepts that a change is warranted, self-efficacy is improved when the patient is able to develop a realistic plan to make the change and then realizes the change is achievable. Self-efficacy will further improve when the patient is able to successfully quit smoking, engage in pulmonary rehabilitation, take medications, and use oxygen and other treatments as prescribed. Pacing, pursed-lip breathing, and the use of aids (e.g., a cane, supplemental oxygen) involve new behaviors that can improve a patient's physical functioning, also improving the patient's feelings of control and confidence. To the extent that patients can exert control and actively manage the disease, they develop more confidence in their ability to do so and are more likely to feel better about themselves and remain motivated to work at coping.

FACTORS THAT INFLUENCE ADJUSTMENT

Although there are few studies on factors that affect adjustment in pulmonary patients, self-efficacy and optimism have both been associated with adjustment in COPD patients (Popa-Velea & Purcarea, 2014). Other personal and external factors can also affect the individual's ability to adjust to a chronic disease. Patients who have good social support, a history of successful coping, and an understanding of the issues they need to address seem to do better with the adjustment process. Conversely, patients with cognitive deficits, poor social support, and few socioeconomic resources will have more difficulty managing the adjustment to their disease. Again, a thorough psychological evaluation will delineate these factors and enable the development of a targeted treatment plan for the individual patient.

6 ANXIETY

Anxiety is common in pulmonary patients, although its severity is variable. Symptoms may be mild and few or may present as a full-blown clinical anxiety disorder. Distinguishing anxiety symptoms that are due to psychological causes from symptoms caused by medical disease or treatment will help determine the appropriate intervention.

PREVALENCE OF ANXIETY IN PULMONARY PATIENTS

Anxiety occurs frequently in patients with chronic lung diseases and is often comorbid with depression (e.g., Yohannes, Kaplan, & Hanania, 2018). In a review of studies with chronic obstructive pulmonary disease (COPD) patients, Willgoss and Yohannes (2013) reported the prevalence of anxiety in inpatients ranged from 10% to 55%, and in outpatients from 13% to 46%. Generalized anxiety disorder occurred in 6% to 33%, with panic disorder in 0% to 41%, specific phobia in 10% to 27%, and social phobia in 5% to 11%. Posttraumatic stress disorder (PTSD) symptoms have also been reported in pulmonary patients as a result of experiences during hospital admissions,

http://dx.doi.org/10.1037/0000189-007
Psychological Treatment of Patients With Chronic Respiratory Disease, by S. M. Labott

and 20% of patients continue to report PTSD symptoms 3 months after a hospital admission (de Miranda et al., 2011).

Similarly, anxiety occurs frequently in other chronic lung diseases such as asthma (36%–45%; e.g., Ciprandi, Schiavetti, Rindone, & Ricciardolo, 2015), cystic fibrosis (CF; 32%; e.g., Quittner et al., 2014), sarcoidosis (33%; Ireland & Wilsher, 2010), and pulmonary fibrosis (21%–31%; e.g., Y. J. Lee et al., 2017). Anxiety and panic occur more frequently in pulmonary patients than in other chronic disease populations, perhaps because of the association of breathlessness with both pulmonary and anxiety disorders (e.g., Del Giacco et al., 2016).

IMPACTS OF ANXIETY IN RESPIRATORY DISEASE

Anxiety has been associated with many negative consequences in pulmonary patients. Studies of patients with COPD (e.g., Yohannes et al., 2018), CF (Yohannes, Willgoss, Fatoye, Dip, & Webb, 2012), and asthma (e.g., Ciprandi et al., 2015) have all noted decreased quality of life in patients with anxiety. Studies of COPD patients have reported an association between anxiety and increased mortality, more frequent symptom exacerbations, worse dyspnea, and increased medical utilization (e.g., Yohannes et al., 2018). In patients with asthma, anxiety and panic are associated with greater perceived dyspnea, more distress over symptoms, and poorer asthma control (e.g., Boudreau et al., 2015; Ciprandi et al., 2015); anxiety is also associated with more severe symptoms in CF (Yohannes et al., 2012). Anxiety is associated with smoking and with increased withdrawal symptoms for pulmonary patients who are attempting to quit smoking (e.g., Yohannes et al., 2018).

CAUSES OF ANXIETY SYMPTOMS

The causes of anxiety in pulmonary patients include premorbid anxiety, new onset anxiety due to a psychological etiology, respiratory disease presenting as anxiety, anxiety symptoms secondary to pulmonary medications, and comorbid anxiety and pulmonary disease. Treatment of the anxiety symptoms will be most effective if the specific cause(s) of the anxiety is delineated and targeted for the individual patient.

Premorbid Anxiety

Patients may present with a preexisting anxiety disorder that was initially unrelated to the lung disease, although, once the lung disease has developed, the anxiety may exacerbate it. An evaluation of the patient's psychological history is important, with a focus on previous psychological treatments. Psychotropic medications will also need to be discussed to determine what has helped the patient to manage the anxiety in the past; these medications may need to be reevaluated (some psychotropics are contraindicated in patients with pulmonary disease).

New Onset Anxiety With a Psychological Etiology

There are many potential causes of anxiety for patients with pulmonary disease. Initially, they may fear the unknown, that is, how the disease may progress and what it may mean for their lives. They may fear specific medical tests (because of anticipated pain or claustrophobia) or the bad news that may follow a medical test. For patients who experience dyspnea, it is common to experience anxiety about shortness of breath recurring. Others are anxious about side effects of medications, the reactions of others if they use oxygen or inhalers in public, and changes to their identity and role in the family.

Patients who report new anxiety and/or posttraumatic stress symptoms following a hospital admission may have recollections of many different types of traumatic experiences (see de Miranda et al., 2011). Some of these are due to the hospital setting itself (e.g., noise, light), to the patient's medical problem (e.g., pain, feelings of suffocation), or perhaps associated with delirium (e.g., fears of being murdered, hallucinations; see Chapter 10 for more on delirium). In short, there are many reasons for new onset anxiety when a patient is dealing with pulmonary disease.

Respiratory Disease Presenting With Anxiety Symptoms

It is not uncommon for patients who are not yet diagnosed with COPD or pulmonary embolus to assume that the shortness of breath they experience is caused by anxiety. Similarly, hyperventilation in an asthma patient may be perceived as anxiety, and these patients may present to a psychologist for treatment. Thorough evaluation will be necessary to determine if the cause of the anxiety symptoms is physiological and caused by the pulmonary disease or whether it is psychological in nature. Psychological treatment alone will have little impact on the symptoms if the underlying respiratory problem is not identified and properly treated.

Anxiety Secondary to Respiratory Medications

Some medications used to treat pulmonary disease are associated with anxiety symptoms, such as bronchodilators (e.g., salmeterol, theophylline) and corticosteroids (e.g., prednisone). When taking these medications, patients may experience tremors, internal jitters (e.g., butterflies in stomach), increased arousal, poor sleep, and increased startle response. In mild cases, an awareness that these experiences are caused by a medication is sufficient for the patient to manage. In severe cases, however, the medication that is causing the symptoms may need to be adjusted or additional medications added to manage these symptoms.

Comorbid Anxiety and Respiratory Disease

The physiological and psychological symptoms may be comorbid and may exacerbate each other, further complicating the picture. Willgoss et al. (2012) described a cycle of anxiety-breathlessness in which either the anxiety symptoms or the respiratory symptoms can cause the other. In the words of a patient:

> It's like a vicious circle. Your breathing gets bad so you get anxious, then you get afraid, and your breathing gets worse, which makes you more afraid. The COPD feeds the anxiety and the anxiety feeds the fear. (Willgoss et al., 2012, p. 565)

Treatment needs to break the cycle: Medical treatment can focus on the physiological causes of the dyspnea, and psychological intervention can target the psychological factors that cause anxiety.

Determining the Cause of the Anxiety Symptoms

An evaluation of the anxiety history and symptoms should be performed, and it should include details on the specific symptoms experienced as well as their onset, duration, triggers, frequency, and strategies to manage them. In conjunction with the evaluation of anxiety symptoms, the patient should be asked about his or her pulmonary history and symptoms, to include specific details of the symptoms experienced, including their onset, duration, and so forth. Patients should be asked about how the anxiety symptoms affect their daily activities, information about strategies that help them manage it, and events that exacerbate it.

Following the interview with the patient, the psychologist will need to sort out the cause(s) of the individual patient's anxiety. In this process, consideration should be given to the history of the anxiety and pulmonary disease, which occurred first historically, and how they relate to each other presently. Triggers of the anxiety symptoms, including life stressors and medications, should be considered, as well as medical treatments or interventions that help the patient to manage the symptoms. The psychologist can then decide on the appropriate treatments, depending on the etiology of the anxiety symptom.

TREATMENT OF ANXIETY IN PULMONARY PATIENTS

Most research on anxiety interventions for patients with pulmonary disease has evaluated multicomponent programs, such as pulmonary rehabilitation programs that may include exercise, education, and relaxation (see reviews by Panagioti, Scott, Blakemore, & Coventry, 2014, and Tselebis et al., 2016). What follows are descriptions of a variety of treatments for anxiety, including education, cognitive behavioral interventions, and psychotropic medications. Although any of these may be helpful as part of a comprehensive treatment program, the outpatient clinician who is treating an individual patient will need to select those components that will provide the most benefit for the specific patient.

Education

Education is often the first-line intervention to manage anxiety in pulmonary patients. Information on the disease itself, the typical course, treatment options, and other relevant information can help patients to feel more in control and better able to manage the disease. (A detailed description of the information to be provided to patients is in Chapter 5.) An understanding of the disease allows patients to develop realistic expectations and decreases catastrophic thinking, thus decreasing anxiety. Similarly, those with traumatic hospital experiences can benefit from education on potential medical causes. Understanding that these experiences are common for hospitalized patients can also help to normalize the experience and increase the expectation of recovery.

Cognitive Behavioral Interventions

A review of randomized controlled trials has reported improvements in quality of life, asthma control, and anxiety in adult asthma patients who received cognitive behavior therapy (Kew, Nashed, Dulay, & Yorke, 2016); reductions in asthma-specific fear have also been reported (Parry et al., 2012). Below are descriptions of several of the more common cognitive behavioral interventions with applications for pulmonary patients. Additional techniques and a case example can be found in Heslop-Marshall (2017).

Cognitive Strategies

Patients may become anxious when experiencing shortness of breath as a result of maladaptive and often catastrophizing cognitions ("Oh no, I can't breathe, this is bad, I could suffocate"), which then further increases the breathlessness. Although patients may be initially unable to articulate cognitions of this sort, they can generally recognize them when asked about them specifically and can then develop an awareness of these cognitions when they occur. Patients can also learn to generate more adaptive cognitions to help promote feelings of mastery and control; for example, "I feel short of breath; what action should I take—use my inhaler, sit down, relax?"; "I know this will pass, I need to remain calm and wait for the medication to work"; "My doctor said this would happen and that I will be OK"; or "This is unpleasant, but I can manage it and it will get easier as I get better at this." Over time and with practice, patients can use these cognitive strategies to cope more effectively with breathlessness when it occurs, avoiding the anxiety-breathlessness spiral (Willgoss et al., 2012). Exhibit 6.1 is a handout

EXHIBIT 6.1. Shortness of Breath Cycle for Chronic Obstructive Pulmonary Disease (COPD) and Asthma

Many people with COPD or asthma experience a shortness of breath cycle. In this cycle, shortness of breath from COPD or asthma leads to worry and panic, which in turn worsens shortness of breath. Here are the steps that often occur: Shortness of breath leads to . . .

- Worry (e.g., about breathing, passing out, dying), leading to . . .
- Anxiety or panic physical reaction, leading to . . .
- Increased breathing rate, leading to . . .
- Less effective (i.e., rapid, shallow) breathing, leading to . . .
- Increased oxygen use by, and less oxygen available for, muscles, leading to . . .
- More shortness of breath . . .
- And the cycle continues.

You can stop the shortness of breath cycle by following these steps:

1. When you first notice shortness of breath, STOP your activity.
2. Rest. Sit down or lie down, if possible.
3. Relax. Use diaphragmatic breathing or pursed-lip breathing techniques.
4. Reassure yourself. Tell yourself reassuring thoughts about your symptoms.
5. If possible, measure and record your peak flow and follow your action plan.
6. Take medications, if appropriate, following your primary care provider's recommendations.
7. After your breathing improves, gradually resume activity in a paced manner.

Note. Reprinted from *Integrated Behavioral Health in Primary Care: Step-by-Step Guidance for Assessment and Intervention* (2nd ed., p. 125), by C. L. Hunter, J. L. Goodie, M. S. Oordt, and A. C. Dobmeyer, 2017, Washington, DC: American Psychological Association. Copyright 2017 by the American Psychological Association.

with education, cognitive, and behavioral strategies for use with patients who struggle with the breathlessness-anxiety cycle.

Relaxation, Breathing, and Imagery
Several methods can be used to promote relaxation in pulmonary patients with anxiety, such as progressive or passive muscle relaxation, diaphragmatic breathing (DB), and imagery. There are also simpler activities that patients can use to relax, such as listening to their favorite music. The goal of any of these strategies is to decrease muscle tension and the frequency of maladaptive cognitions for patients who are anxious or who have intrusive memories following a hospital admission. In patients with COPD, relaxation has been shown to reduce feelings of anxiety and dyspnea (Singh, Rao, Prem, Sahoo, & Keshav, 2009) and to increase feelings of well-being (Volpato, Banfi, Rogers, & Pagnini, 2015). Biofeedback has been shown to decrease anxiety generally (e.g., Goessl, Curtiss, & Hofmann, 2017), although little research has been done in the pulmonary population.

The patient's medical situation should be taken into account when choosing a relaxation procedure. Progressive muscle relaxation is generally not the best technique for those with moderate-severe pulmonary disease, because the muscle tension involves exertion and could tire patients and increase shortness of breath. In this situation, passive relaxation is more appropriate as patients are asked to focus on muscles and relax them, without tensing them first.

DB is often a good strategy, although many patients are already familiar with pursed-lip breathing and will find it easier to use that, rather than learning a new procedure. (For those unfamiliar with pursed-lip breathing, Hunter, Goodie, Oordt, & Dobmeyer, 2017, p. 130, provided a handout describing its effects, as well as how and when to use it.) Although DB and pursed-lip breathing can be used with patients on supplemental oxygen, they should not be used for patients on a ventilator, because the vent is guiding the patient's breathing and the patient should not try to override that. On occasion, a patient may become more anxious when focusing on diaphragmatic breathing; if that occurs, another relaxation strategy should be used.

Imagery can be useful for all; a version of guided imagery in which people imagined themselves relaxed in a nice place was the most preferred of six relaxation strategies in a group of COPD patients (Hyland et al., 2016). Basic relaxation and DB techniques are found in Bourne (2015); imagery is described in Labott (2019).

Distraction
Although most people know of activities that they can use to distract themselves, they may not think of using them to cope with anxiety. People can

read, socialize with family and friends, watch television, or work on hobbies to distract themselves from the worries that escalate anxiety. They may need to be encouraged to actively seek activities that distract them when they experience anxiety.

Desensitization

Sleep apnea is a disorder in which people stop breathing while they sleep. The medical treatment is to provide pressure to the airway to keep it from closing, usually using continuous positive airway pressure (CPAP), which requires the patient to wear a mask or nasal pillows (inserts for the nose, similar to ear plugs for swimming) when sleeping. Some patients feel anxious or claustrophobic and are unable to tolerate wearing a mask; nasal pillows are often easier to tolerate. Nonadherence to the CPAP treatment occurs in 30% to 60% of patients (Rotenberg, Murariu, & Pang, 2016). This is a significant problem because untreated sleep apnea causes sleep deprivation that is associated with many negative consequences, such as headaches, snoring, cognitive changes, hypoxemia (that can cause tissue damage), cardiovascular mortality, and daytime hypersomnolence that causes automobile or other accidents (e.g., Chaudhary et al., 2016; Weinberger et al., 2019). Desensitization can be useful to help patients to tolerate the intervention, aiding compliance. It is often paired with education and cognitive strategies.

Initially, patients are reeducated about the importance of the CPAP treatment for their health and misunderstandings are clarified. For example, some patients report anxiety because they fear they will suffocate if the electricity fails and the machine turns off. They are often able to tolerate this treatment if they understand that they will not suffocate—they will simply wake up and take the mask off.

For patients who are claustrophobic about wearing the mask, it is useful to do a desensitization procedure in which the patient interacts with the machine (rather than through imagery) after learning to use relaxation strategies. As in any desensitization procedure, patients learn to proceed from less anxiety-provoking events to more anxiety-provoking events using relaxation to remain calm. Sample items in a desensitization hierarchy could include examining the parts of the device, listening to the sound the machine makes, holding the mask against the face, wearing the mask with the machine turned off, holding the mask near the face with the air flowing, strapping the mask on briefly, and wearing the mask for longer periods of time. The speed with which people progress through the steps will depend on the severity of the anxiety, but improvement typically occurs in only a few sessions.

Interoceptive Exposure Treatments

Much anxiety treatment, such as the desensitization procedure described previously, is based on exposing the individual to the feared stimuli. Interoceptive exposure (see Boettcher, Brake, & Barlow, 2016) has also been used to help individuals manage anxiety associated with unpleasant physical sensations, such as shortness of breath or pain. However, if symptoms such as shortness of breath or hyperventilation are induced in a patient with pulmonary disease, and if they are intense enough, they could trigger serious respiratory problems that could pose a danger to the patient. Therefore, anxiety treatment strategies that will not tax the patient's respiratory system are preferred.

Psychotropic Medication

The Global Initiative for Chronic Obstructive Lung Disease (GOLD; 2018) guidelines indicate that anxiety can be treated in patients with COPD as it would be in any patient without respiratory disease. However, benzodiazepines can decrease respiratory drive and may also cause carbon dioxide retention, creating potentially serious respiratory side effects in patients with severe respiratory disease (e.g., Battaglia, Bezzi, & Sferrazza Papa, 2014; Ford & Wheaton, 2015). Therefore, benzodiazepines should be used cautiously in patients with respiratory disease. Buspirone can also be used to treat anxiety in respiratory patients, but it is less practical because it can take several weeks for patients to experience the beneficial effects (Colón & Popkin, 2002).

In summary, there are many causes of anxiety in pulmonary patients, as well as overlap between pulmonary and anxiety symptoms and comorbid presentations. Although these anxiety management strategies are frequently used with outpatients, there are also inpatient applications for patients with acute illness. Case 6.1 presents a case in which imagery and distraction were used to decrease anxiety while the inpatient was being weaned from a ventilator. Regardless of the setting, intervention will be most effective if the cause(s) is delineated and the specific treatment components target that cause.

CASE 6.1
ANXIETY ASSOCIATED WITH VENTILATOR WEANING

The psychologist, Dr. S, was consulted to see a hospitalized patient with idiopathic pulmonary fibrosis (IPF) who was admitted with pneumonia and had been on a ventilator for 10 days. The patient's physician planned to start weaning the patient (Mrs. M) from the vent within the next few days, and the patient was quite anxious that she would not be able to breathe without it.

Dr. S reviewed the patient's medical record and saw Mrs. M the next morning. She was a 64 y/o woman who had been diagnosed with IPF several years ago, and she was stable medically until she developed recent pneumonia. The patient was awake and alert at the evaluation and was aware of the weaning plans. She had a history of mild anxiety, had been in outpatient psychotherapy, and knew how to use diaphragmatic breathing.

The treatment plan was to provide the patient with strategies that she could learn quickly to help her successfully tolerate the weaning process over the next few days. These included (a) providing education, (b) reminding the patient she is in control of the process, (c) teaching her to use imagery to relax, and (d) developing distraction plans to decrease her focus on the weaning. Dr. S explained she would provide the patient with strategies to help her successfully wean off the vent. She reminded the patient of the benefits of being independent of the ventilator and reviewed the procedures that Mrs. M's doctors and nurses had discussed with her. Specifically, the patient was reminded that the vent would be turned down (*not off*) so that it would provide her with less breathing support. The patient's oxygen saturation and subjective feelings of breathlessness would be checked by her nurse every 15 minutes. If the patient's oxygen saturation was OK, and if she felt comfortable, after about an hour the vent would be turned down further and the same process followed. This would go on for a few hours each day for a few days, until Mrs. M was able to breathe comfortably on her own, without any ventilator support.

Dr. S explained that Mrs. M was in control of the process so that if, at any time, she felt unable to breathe and wanted to end the trial, her nurse would stop it. Training on techniques (e.g., imagery, distraction) to help the patient manage her anxiety was suggested, and the patient agreed. Dr. S then helped the patient to select a relaxing event (Vivaldi's *The Four Seasons* played by her local symphony orchestra) and guided the patient through an imagery exercise in which she was encouraged to relax and to imagine herself in a park near her home. She was guided to first experience spring, with trees and flowers beginning to bud, and the warm breeze and birds singing. Imagery was provided for each of the four seasons. The patient seemed to

CASE 6.1

ANXIETY ASSOCIATED WITH VENTILATOR WEANING
(*Continued*)

physically relax and reported the most benefit from the summer imagery, so this was chosen as her primary image, and she agreed to practice it again later in the day on her own.

Distraction was also discussed, as well as the negative consequences of focusing on her breathing during the weaning trial (i.e., it would make it more difficult). Mrs. M agreed to collect some activities to help her to distract herself when the weaning trial began (e.g., a mystery she was reading, a cooking podcast, crossword puzzles).

The next day Dr. S arrived to see the patient shortly after the weaning trial had begun. The patient was mildly anxious but was doing OK. They practiced the imagery for about 20 minutes and Mrs. M was able to decrease her anxiety a bit more. Afterward she also felt more confident that she would be able to successfully wean from the ventilator. She had her distraction materials and planned to keep herself busy throughout the trial. Overall, the patient was able to manage and continue with the weaning process. Her sister arrived to visit with her (providing both support and distraction) so the psychologist left with plans to return the next day.

The following day the weaning trial was again underway when the psychologist arrived. The patient was again mildly anxious but proudly reported that the previous day's trial had gone on for almost two hours and that she had done well. She had not experienced much shortness of breath, but she was physically and emotionally tired after the trial. She noted a few episodes of mild to moderate anxiety and reported that the distraction strategies had worked well, but she had trouble maintaining the imagery. The psychologist again provided the guided imagery and the patient did well with it. She was comfortable continuing on her own through today's weaning trial. Again, while some strategies were more successful than others, the patient was able to sufficiently manage her anxiety to allow her to continue weaning without significant distress.

The next day the psychologist again came to see the patient and was pleased to see that the weaning had been successful and Mrs. M was no longer receiving ventilator support. The psychologist reviewed the strategies that had helped the patient manage her anxiety during the weaning process and also discussed other situations in which Mrs. M could use these to manage anxiety in her life generally.

7 DEPRESSION

Depression is common in patients with pulmonary disease and is often comorbid with anxiety (see Chapter 6); patients may experience only a few mild symptoms to a severe major depressive episode. Any symptoms of depression or changes in mood can create problems for patients with pulmonary disease and, therefore, warrant attention.

PREVALENCE AND IMPACTS OF DEPRESSION IN LUNG DISEASE

The chronic obstructive pulmonary disease (COPD) literature reports depression in 10% to 42% of patients with stable COPD, and in 10% to 86% of those experiencing COPD exacerbations (e.g., Yohannes, Kaplan, & Hanania, 2018). Depression occurs in those with COPD at a higher rate than healthy matched controls (18.8% vs. 3.5%; Di Marco et al., 2006), and there is a greater risk of depression in patients with COPD than in patients with other chronic illnesses (Cuijpers et al., 2014). Patients with severe COPD are twice as likely to be depressed as those with milder COPD (Yohannes et al., 2018).

http://dx.doi.org/10.1037/0000189-008
Psychological Treatment of Patients With Chronic Respiratory Disease, by S. M. Labott

Depression also occurs frequently in other chronic respiratory disorders. In cystic fibrosis (CF), depression has been reported in 17% to 19% of patients (e.g., Quittner et al., 2014). Borson and Curtis (2001) have reported that 60% of the patients in their sample with sarcoidosis screened positive for depression, although rates in sarcoidosis (e.g., Ireland & Wilsher, 2010), asthma (Labor, Labor, Jurić, & Vuksić, 2012), and idiopathic pulmonary fibrosis (Y. J. Lee et al., 2017) are generally around 25%. Lowe et al. (2004) reported 15.9% of patients with pulmonary hypertension had major depressive disorder.

Much of the research on the role of depression in pulmonary disease has been completed with COPD patients. These studies have reported that depression is associated with increased mortality, more frequent exacerbations and hospitalizations, increased dyspnea, poorer adherence, decreased quality of life, and decreased functional capacity (Ouellette & Lavoie, 2017; Yohannes et al., 2018). Decreased quality of life is associated with depression in CF (Yohannes, Willgoss, Fatoye, Dip, & Webb, 2012) and pulmonary hypertension (Harzheim et al., 2013). Decreased lung function is associated with depression in CF (Yohannes et al., 2012). Although the measures and populations used in these studies varied, the results overwhelmingly demonstrate that depression occurs frequently in chronic lung disease and that it has negative effects.

COPD is a risk factor for suicide; a recent review reported that "a person with COPD is 90% more likely to commit suicide than a person without COPD" (Sampaio et al., 2019, p. 16). In this review, the risk of suicide was associated with factors such as depression, quality of life, age, and substance use. Hospitalizations have been shown to increase the risk for suicide in COPD patients, even when the contribution of psychological illness is removed (Strid, Christiansen, Olsen, & Qin, 2014). The studies of depression and suicide highlight the importance of attention to these issues when evaluating and treating pulmonary patients.

CAUSES OF DEPRESSION IN CHRONIC LUNG DISEASE PATIENTS

Patients may develop lung disease in the context of a premorbid depression, or they may develop new symptoms of depression associated with limitations imposed by the lung disease. Pulmonary diseases and depression share certain characteristics, and each can cause or exacerbate the other.

Premorbid Depression

Depression that predates the lung disease may have developed as a result of totally unrelated problems, but it can still influence the course of the lung disease. Psychomotor symptoms that are due to depression can exacerbate the physical symptoms of the lung disease, and premorbid depression can affect the patient's ability and motivation to adhere to the medical treatment regimen. For patients with premorbid depression, the clinician will want to do a thorough assessment of the psychological history and current treatment to ensure that a patient's ongoing psychological or psychiatric treatment is not overlooked.

New Onset Depression

It is easy to see how patients with chronic lung disease could develop depression; in patients newly diagnosed with COPD, new onset depression was 88% higher than in matched controls (Yohannes & Alexopoulos, 2014a). As the disease progresses, patients may experience losses that result from severe dyspnea, the need for supplemental oxygen, or physical limitations. People may be unable to work or participate in hobbies and social activities; this can result in changes in the patient's role at home or work. Changes to their self-esteem and identity can also occur. Additional medical problems such as heart disease, cancer, or tumor necrosis alpha (which is associated with inflammation) can exacerbate the patient's medical problems and associated losses. People with comorbidities will have a greater burden in terms of health care, more difficulty maintaining their quality of life, and, perhaps, more worry about the future and what it holds.

Risk factors for depression in chronic lung disease also include social factors; people with lower socioeconomic status have fewer resources available to them, and those who are socially isolated have less support. Cognitive problems make all this more difficult for patients, and they may require that patients depend heavily on others, losing their independence. Those with low self-esteem may have more difficulty coping. Gender and age can also play a role in the development of depression. Many patients face a constellation of risk factors including the development of a progressive disease, social isolation due to retirement or the loss of a spouse, and new cognitive and physical limitations. Some patients will actively take on the challenges and successfully adjust to their medical situation, whereas others can develop hopelessness and other symptoms of depression that can endure. Exhibit 7.1 is a list of factors that are associated with depression in COPD and asthma patients.

EXHIBIT 7.1. Association of Physical and Socioeconomic Factors With Occurrence of Depression in Patients With Chronic Obstructive Pulmonary Disease (COPD) and Asthma

Increased physical disability
Severity of COPD or asthma
Social isolation
Severe dyspnea
Older age
Female gender
Impaired quality of life
Lower socioeconomic status
Low self-esteem
Decreased exercise tolerance
Being on long-term oxygen therapy
Cognitive impairment
Tumor necrosis alpha
Presence of two or more comorbidities

Note. From "The Impact of Depression in Older Patients With Chronic Obstructive Pulmonary Disease and Asthma," by M. J. Connolly and A. M. Yohannes, 2016, *Maturitas, 92*, p. 10. Copyright 2016 by Elsevier. Reprinted with permission.

Overlap of Lung Disease and Depressive Symptoms

Some symptoms of lung disease overlap with those of depression, and this can cause problems in the patient's treatment if the psychologist is unaware of the role of pulmonary disease. For example, if a patient presents to an outpatient psychologist complaining of low energy, poor sleep, decreased activity, and poor appetite, the psychologist may diagnose depression. Yet any or all of these symptoms can be due to the lung disease, and, conversely, depression may not be present at all.

In general, the medications used to treat pulmonary disease are not associated with the development of depression. One exception is corticosteroids. As noted in Chapter 6, corticosteroids are associated with anxiety symptoms, but side effects also include mood disorders and depression (e.g., Kenna, Poon, de los Angeles, & Koran, 2011). It is important that a thorough biopsychosocial evaluation defines the pulmonary, medication, and psychological issues, because psychological treatment will be most effective when targeting symptoms that are responsive to psychological techniques.

Bidirectional Nature of Lung Disease and Depression

As noted earlier, there are many studies demonstrating that depression is associated with negative outcomes in chronic lung disease patients. In a review of studies with COPD patients, Atlantis, Fahey, Cochrane, and Smith

(2013) also demonstrated that COPD increases the risk of depression. That is, patients with COPD had a 55% to 69% increased risk of developing depression.

The mechanisms associated with this bidirectional relationship are unclear. There is evidence that depression can result in nonadherence, creating worse pulmonary symptoms and poorer prognosis (e.g., Atlantis et al., 2013). Increased dyspnea and decreased exercise capacity caused by the lung disease are also associated with both anxiety and depression (Tetikkurt et al., 2011). Persistent smoking is associated with depression (see Rzadkiewicz, Bråtas, & Espnes, 2016) and also has significant negative implications for the lung disease (Weinberger et al., 2019). Finally, it has been hypothesized that inflammation mediates the relationship between depressive symptoms and pulmonary function (Yohannes et al., 2018).

DETECTING DEPRESSION IN PULMONARY PATIENTS

Even though depression is fairly common in patients with lung disease, it is often undetected and not treated. Only half of depressed patients are accurately diagnosed in primary care (Simon, 2002), and of those diagnosed with depression or anxiety, only 31% received treatment to address those psychological symptoms (Kunik et al., 2005).

To address this problem, Maurer et al. (2008) recommended that physicians use brief screening questions to assess for symptoms of depression (and other psychological symptoms). The Patient Health Questionnaire–9 (PHQ-9; https://www.phqscreeners.com/select-screener/) is a commonly used measure for this purpose and is shown in Exhibit 7.2. The Patient Health Questionnaire–2 (PHQ-2; also at https://www.phqscreeners.com/select-screener/) is even shorter and consists of the first two items of the PHQ-9. Items are scored 0 (*not at all*) to 3 (*nearly every day*). Several suggestions for evaluating responses are provided on the website, but a score of 10 or higher on the PHQ-9 warrants additional evaluation (e.g., a more extensive assessment through either additional testing or psychological interview, or both) or intervention. Yohannes et al. (2018) described several other useful screening measures for depression and anxiety. The psychologist may want to recommend that physicians use screeners such as these and can provide information on what score should prompt a referral to a mental health professional.

Maurer et al. (2008) reviewed a variety of barriers to pulmonary patients receiving treatment for depression. Specifically, these authors described

EXHIBIT 7.2. Patient Health Questionnaire-9

Over the last 2 weeks, how often have you been bothered by any of the following problems (*not at all, several days, more than half the days,* or *nearly every day*)?

1. Little interest or pleasure in doing things
2. Feeling down, depressed, or hopeless
3. Trouble falling or staying asleep, or sleeping too much
4. Feeling tired or having little energy
5. Poor appetite or overeating
6. Feeling bad about yourself—or that you are a failure or have let yourself or your family down
7. Trouble concentrating on things, such as reading the newspaper or watching television
8. Moving or speaking so slowly that other people could have noticed? Or the opposite—being so fidgety or restless that you have been moving around a lot more than usual
9. Thoughts that you would be better off dead or of hurting yourself in some way

Note. Reprinted from the *Patient Health Questionnaire (PHQ) Screeners,* by R. L. Spitzer, J. B. W. Williams, K. Kroenke, et al., n.d., Pfizer (https://www.phqscreeners.com/select-screener/). In the public domain.

patient-level barriers that interfere with depression detection and treatment, including a lack of knowledge about depression and treatment options, stigma about mental illness, a lack of available treatment options and mental health coverage, reluctance to disclose symptoms, and a masking of mood symptoms by the physical symptoms. They also described physician-level barriers, such as a lack of a standardized approach to the diagnosis of psychological problems, decreased use of screening questionnaires, a lack of confidence or skill in the psychological assessment, minimal time to spend with patients, and a decreased ability to monitor adherence and outcomes. Finally, system-level barriers also interfere with depression treatment, including a lack of medical records, poor communication between primary care physicians and mental health professionals, an emphasis on productivity rather than time with patients, and poor insurance for mental health treatment.

To address these problems, Katon, Von Korff, Lin, and Simon (2001) described a collaborative-care model in which another professional (e.g., a nurse) works with the primary care physician to educate patients and to monitor adherence and outcomes. In addition, a specialist (presumably a psychologist or psychiatrist) consults with the primary team on the depression treatment. This model has been associated with improved depression treatment and also improved patient outcomes (Maurer et al., 2008).

More recently, Dobmeyer (2018) described the primary care behavioral health (PCBH) model in which a behavioral health consultant collaborates with the primary care team to educate, provide clinical services to patients, and work with the primary care team to improve their assessment and intervention skills. Research has demonstrated that the use of the PCBH model results in decreases in depression symptoms, improved follow-up with behavioral health appointments, and increased patient and provider satisfaction (Dobmeyer, 2018).

Although designed for primary care clinics, the principles and practices of the PCBH model can easily be applied to a pulmonary specialty clinic in which a psychologist is present to assess and intervene with patients presenting with psychological symptoms, educate patients and staff about psychological symptoms and interventions, and connect patients with more intensive psychological or psychiatric services, if warranted. Dobmeyer (2018) described how the PCBH model could be implemented with asthma patients in primary care.

INTERVENTION

There are a variety of useful interventions for depression in chronic pulmonary patients, including education, cognitive behavioral techniques, and medication. Pulmonary rehabilitation, a multidisciplinary approach, incorporates components of any or all of these.

Psychoeducation

As noted throughout this book, education is an important part not only of the medical treatment of lung disease but also of psychological intervention. Patients need to be educated about the potential causes and specific symptoms of depression. Many patients see depression as "a bad day" and do not understand the variety of symptoms that can be associated with it. They also need to understand that depression is evaluated on the basis of the number of symptoms experienced, as well as their intensity and duration, and that anything from a mild depressed mood to a severe clinical depression may warrant attention. They should be aware that these symptoms occur frequently in patients with lung disease for many reasons and that it is important to monitor themselves for the presence and severity of depressive symptoms.

Pulmonary patients need to understand the overlap between depression and pulmonary symptoms and be encouraged to learn to differentiate them. That is, if a patient is reticent to attend a family gathering, is the reluctance the result of decreased physical energy and dyspnea associated with the required physical activity, or is it caused by decreased motivation and interest secondary to depression, or is it some combination of those factors? It may take time, but most patients are able to learn to distinguish the pulmonary from the psychological symptoms; knowing the cause will help them decide what they need to do to proceed in the most adaptive manner.

Care should be taken to avoid patients getting the impression that they are psychiatric patients if they experience symptoms of depression. Rather, they should understand that many of these reactions are expected because of the disease they are dealing with, but that these symptoms can and should be addressed to improve their overall quality of life and functioning. Patients can also be educated about treatments for depression, certainly in more detail if they are or have experienced symptoms. They should also be provided with information on whom to contact if symptoms worsen or if they develop additional symptoms. Education of this sort gives patients a perspective from which to view the symptoms, as well as direction regarding the appropriate response.

Cognitive Behavior Therapy

Cognitive behavior therapy (CBT; Beck, Rush, Shaw, & Emery, 1979) is known as an effective treatment for depression generally (e.g., Powers, de Kleine, & Smits, 2017). Although there is no reason to expect that CBT would be less effective with pulmonary patients, only a few trials have been done with CBT in this population. Studies and reviews have noted small but positive effects of CBT (e.g., Ouellette & Lavoie, 2017; Smith, Sonego, Ketcheson, & Larson, 2014). Studies tend to show small decreases in depression symptoms, but many were methodologically poor, and the CBT interventions did not always contain the same components (e.g., relaxation, cognitive therapy, education, self-management training). More recently, Alexopoulos et al. (2016) provided a treatment designed to motivate patients to participate actively in their medical treatment with or without problem-solving skills training. Results indicated that both treatments resulted in clinically important decreases in depression in over 70% of patients.

Thus far, there is no manualized CBT treatment for pulmonary patients. Psychologists treating depression in this group will need to tailor the treatment to the individual patient, focusing on problems such as social isolation, poor self-esteem, and other factors associated with depression in chronic lung patients. Several of these treatment components are described below.

Restructuring Maladaptive Cognitions

Cognitive approaches to depression target maladaptive cognitions to decrease symptoms of depression and promote more adaptive behavior. (Basic techniques can be found in Beck et al., 1979.) Cognitive interventions can target the patient's appraisal of physical limitations that are due to the lung disease, mastery and control over the pulmonary symptoms, as well as expectations for the future. Patients can learn to combat hopelessness by accurately evaluating both their current situation and their future prognosis, using data from their doctors and their own experiences. They can learn to evaluate their own ability to manage symptoms properly (as well as areas in which they need more skill). As with any cognitive therapy for depression, patients can learn to challenge cognitions that are associated with depressed mood.

Activity Scheduling

One of the mainstays of depression treatment (Beck et al., 1979), activity scheduling can be an important component of treatment for pulmonary patients. Generally, the treatment involves helping patients to become more physically and socially active; this can increase social reinforcement, create personal feelings of well-being, and decrease rumination. In the context of chronic lung disease, the specifics of the activities may need to be adjusted, depending on the severity of the patient's disease; patients with significant limitations will not be able to engage in activities to the same degree as a person without severe pulmonary disease. For these patients, activity should be broadly defined to include those that involve minimal or no exertion. For example, for a patient with severe dyspnea, rather than attending a dinner out and a basketball game with friends, the adapted activity could include friends bringing a carry-out dinner and spending time with the patient at home. Similarly, rather than playing catch with his grandson, a patient with COPD may spend time with his grandson playing video games. Regardless of the specific activities chosen, the goals are to keep the patient active cognitively, socially, and physically (to the extent that physical activity is safe and well tolerated by the patient).

Pleasant Event Scheduling

Many patients with chronic lung disease are unable to engage in much physical activity and may spend a significant amount of time managing the disease (e.g., using inhalers, getting prescription refills, attending doctor appointments and pulmonary rehabilitation). They may report no energy to do anything else, and they may be physically unable to engage in the activities that brought them joy prior to the development of the lung disease. Patients may struggle to find positive events in which they are able to engage, but they can be encouraged to consider new activities that can provide pleasure, for example, reading a new book, having coffee at their favorite coffee shop, having a long phone call with an old friend, or feeding wild birds. A list of potentially pleasant events provided by Lewinsohn and Graf (1973) can be used to help patients think more broadly about activities that can bring them pleasure. They may then need to be encouraged to work these pleasurable activities into their schedule on a regular basis.

Exercise

Also known for its effects on depression, the exercise component of pulmonary rehabilitation (PR) programs is likely somewhat responsible for improvements in depression for participants (see below). Patients may need help from a psychologist to adhere to a PR program, or they may need to develop plans to initiate and maintain an independent exercise program. Whereas some patients are able to do this on their own, others may need formal plans regarding the timing and duration of exercise, reinforcement for meeting goals, and plans to promote adherence. Some patients may not have PR available to them; after appropriate evaluation and recommendations from the patient's doctor, the psychologist may then help the patient to develop plans to include exercise in his daily routine.

Pacing

Patients may overdo their physical activity, especially on days they feel good, but then they may suffer with increased fatigue later. Pacing involves people engaging in physical activities (e.g., household chores) in ways that allow them to accomplish the task while keeping their level of exertion and breathlessness at a minimal level. This can be done either by scheduling work and breaks on the basis of time segments (i.e., 15 minutes of chores, then 10 minutes of rest) or by natural breaks in the task (e.g., when making dinner: peel carrots, short break, peel potatoes, short break, prepare and place meat in oven). Pacing such as this can help patients to accomplish the desired task successfully and comfortably, but it takes practice to determine how much time should be spent on tasks and breaks, which will be specific to an individual patient. Patients will need to allow more time than usual for the task so they can avoid hurrying, which can result in breathlessness.

There are other tips that can be provided to patients to allow them to function more comfortably, such as to place frequently used dishes at midbody level in the kitchen to avoid reaching overhead, or to invest in a shower chair so that they can sit in the shower. An occupational therapist can provide additional suggestions of this sort. Any of these behavioral techniques can be a part of an intervention program to address depression symptoms and quality of life.

Case 7.1 describes a pulmonary patient with anxiety and depression who was treated with CBT. Heslop-Marshall (2017) offers another example, with a description of the specific CBT techniques used in that case.

CASE 7.1

COGNITIVE BEHAVIOR THERAPY FOR DEPRESSION AND ANXIETY SYMPTOMS

Background

Mrs. B is a 68-year-old woman with COPD, referred by her pulmonologist with concerns about depression and anxiety. She also has hypercholesterolemia, controlled with a statin. Patient lives alone and generally does well. She has two married sons and three grandkids. One of her sons stops by weekly to check on her and she talks with each of them by phone every few days. Patient is a retired kindergarten teacher.

She is recently discharged from the hospital after an admission for pneumonia. She had begun coughing and was short of breath. Over a few days her symptoms worsened, and she became weak. Her cognition became mildly impaired (likely due to infection and decreased oxygenation), and it was not certain that she was taking her medication as prescribed (although generally her adherence had been good). Patient's son noticed these changes and brought her to the hospital.

Patient has no previous psychiatric history—no psychotropic medications, no hospital admissions, no outpatient treatment. No drug or alcohol problems past or current. Since the hospital admission she reports feeling down, and she experiences anxiety symptoms if she becomes dyspneic. She has stopped walking the three blocks to her church for services, bingo, and other activities.

Evaluation

Patient acknowledges depressed mood, sleep is OK, appetite down since pneumonia but improving slowly, no suicidal ideation, no guilt, no worthlessness, no hopelessness or helplessness, decreased motivation and energy. Anxiety symptoms are new, secondary to breathlessness, and she is afraid shortness of breath could progress to a major problem and she

(continues)

CASE 7.1

COGNITIVE BEHAVIOR THERAPY FOR DEPRESSION AND ANXIETY SYMPTOMS (*Continued*)

will suffocate. She also feels her heart rate increase, and she worries about the occurrence of future episodes of anxiety. No generalized anxiety or panic, no hallucinations or delusions. No subjective memory problems. On exam, patient was alert and oriented × 3 (not date). Registration, attention, short- and long-term memory intact. Speech is normal in rate and rhythm. Mood is mildly depressed.

Conceptualization

Patient with no formal psychological history prior to the recent pneumonia. She currently is experiencing new onset depressed mood, as she has experienced new medical problems and physical limitations due to COPD. She also now experiences anxiety associated with breathlessness, as well as anticipatory anxiety. She has limited her physical activity, so she no longer walks to church several times weekly; this has also decreased her social contact and support.

Treatment Plan

After biopsychosocial evaluation, the plan below was developed with the patient; each of the numbered topics were generally explained to her, as well as the rationale for how each could help her to manage her disease, as well as the symptoms of anxiety and depression.

1. Education
   a. Teach patient about anxiety and depression and their occurrence in COPD
   b. Educate patient's sons about medical and psychological symptoms to monitor

2. Determine how much activity is safe
   a. Get doctor's input on amount of physical activity that is safe
   b. Check with nurse practitioner about getting Mrs. B into a PR program
   c. Patient to self-monitor activity and breathlessness to learn her limitations

3. Increase activity
   a. Patient to engage in activities consistent with #2 above; avoid restricting activities unnecessarily
   b. If patient needs to give up an activity because it is too difficult physically, she should find another activity (that requires less exertion) to replace it

CASE 7.1

COGNITIVE BEHAVIOR THERAPY FOR DEPRESSION AND ANXIETY SYMPTOMS (*Continued*)

    c. Family to visit more, adolescent kids to see patient after school for homework

    d. Enlist someone to drive her to church activities

4. Cognitive behavioral strategies for anxiety management

    a. Patient to learn cognitive strategies to decrease her anxiety when she is short of breath

    b. Patient also to learn relaxation techniques to help calm herself when anxious

Outcome

Patient was seen for 6 weeks of psychotherapy. Each of the issues above was addressed with a focus on the specific points listed above. The patient participated in appropriate homework and skill-building exercises. The nurse practitioner was able to get Mrs. B enrolled in PR near her home, and she attended twice weekly. In the PR program she learned additional ways to manage her disease and also began to develop new and supportive relationships. Her family became more engaged, and the patient received additional instrumental and emotional support from her sons, and she enjoyed spending more time with her grandchildren. Mrs. B's mood improved. She still became anxious when she became short of breath, but the symptoms were less intense and she was able to manage them successfully (using the cognitive techniques and relaxation). Patient was scheduled for three more sessions at 6-week intervals, to be sure she was able to maintain these gains. She was encouraged to call the psychologist for additional follow-up as needed.

Pulmonary Rehabilitation

PR is a comprehensive program that is primarily focused on exercise but may also include education, behavioral techniques, and adherence coaching. (See Tucker and Stoermer [2017] for a description of PR program elements as well as a case study.) Several researchers have reported reductions in depressive symptoms for patients participating in PR (e.g., Maurer et al., 2008; Yohannes & Alexopoulos, 2014a). Although the psychologist would not be the primary service provider in PR, she or he can work as part of a multidisciplinary team, offering education, behavioral strategies, techniques to improve adherence and social support, and other psychological interventions that, as part of the larger PR program, can influence depression and the patient's overall quality of life.

Medication

Global Initiative for Chronic Obstructive Lung Disease (GOLD; 2018) recommendations indicate that treatment for depression in patients with COPD should be no different than treatment for depression in anyone else. The choice of a medication should depend on the specific depression symptom profile, potential side effects, as well as possible interactions with nonpsychotropic medications (Tselebis et al., 2016). In general, antidepressants do not affect respiratory drive, although some can be problematic for patients with hypercapnia (carbon dioxide retention; Tselebis et al., 2016). The main categories of medications used for depression in pulmonary patients are selective serotonin reuptake inhibitors (SSRIs) and tricyclic antidepressants (TCAs); SSRIs are often the first line of treatment because they are associated with fewer side effects. (Cruz, Marciel, Quittner, & Schechter, 2009, have noted that the weight gain associated with SSRIs may be of benefit in patients with CF.) Only a few studies have been performed on the use of SSRIs and TCAs in pulmonary patients; some have noted improvements in depression, but there are also conflicting reports (e.g., Pollok, van Agteren, & Carson-Chahhoud, 2018; Yohannes & Alexopoulos, 2014b).

The severity of the depression will determine the intensity or the number of interventions (or both) prescribed for the patient. Thus far, there is evidence for the efficacy of CBT and PR for the treatment of depression, perhaps because these interventions include multiple components, such as education and behavioral techniques. There is less evidence for the efficacy of psychotropic medication for the treatment of depression in patients with chronic lung disease.

8 TOBACCO AND OTHER INHALED SUBSTANCES

Tobacco use is unfortunately common; in 2017, 14% of adults in the United States, or 34.3 million people, smoked cigarettes (Centers for Disease Control and Prevention [CDC], 2019b). People also smoke or inhale other substances that cause respiratory symptoms and diseases. Cessation of the use of these substances is key, and a variety of methods are available to accomplish this.

RESPIRATORY EFFECTS OF SMOKING TOBACCO AND OTHER SUBSTANCES

Tobacco smoking is well known as the "dominant cause of COPD [chronic obstructive pulmonary disease]" in the United States (U.S. Department of Health & Human Services, 2014) and is implicated in 80% to 90% of diagnoses of COPD (Wagena, Huibers, & van Schayck, 2001). The prevalence of COPD among adults in the United States who are current, former, or never smokers is 15.2%, 7.6%, and 2.8%, respectively (Wheaton et al., 2019). Smoking tobacco is associated with increased lung symptoms, decreased

http://dx.doi.org/10.1037/0000189-009
Psychological Treatment of Patients With Chronic Respiratory Disease, by S. M. Labott

lung functioning, greater decline in FEV_1 (forced expiratory volume in 1 second; see Chapter 2), and greater mortality in patients with COPD (e.g., Bai, Chen, Liu, Yu, & Xu, 2017; Global Initiative for Chronic Obstructive Lung Disease [GOLD], 2018). Smoking tobacco exacerbates asthma in adults and likely plays a role in causing the development of asthma initially (U.S. Department of Health & Human Services, 2014). Smoking increases the risk of developing tuberculosis (TB) and is associated with increased mortality and recurrent TB infection (Jeyashree, Kathirvel, Shewade, Kaur, & Goel, 2016). The tar and other chemicals inhaled when smoking cigarettes causes physical harm to the individual; although nicotine is addictive, the nicotine itself does not cause the lung damage associated with smoking (Agrawal & Britton, 2017).

Water-pipe smoking (WPS) involves inhaling vapor that is passed through water. The device for this mode of delivery is known as a *hookah*. Flavored tobacco is usually smoked, although marijuana and opium can also be smoked in this way. Several studies have documented that WPS decreases lung functioning and increases the risk of chronic lung disease (e.g., Raad et al., 2011), likely because people are usually smoking tobacco, simply using a different method. In a typical hookah session, an individual may inhale 100 to 200 times more smoke than in a cigarette (Food and Drug Administration, 2018). In 2018, 2.6 million people used "pipes, water pipes, or hookahs" (Wang et al., 2018).

Marijuana is a commonly used drug that is often smoked. In 2018, 43.5 million Americans over age 12 had used marijuana in the past year, and its use has increased over the past 15 years (Substance Abuse and Mental Health Services Administration, 2019a). Several studies have documented that respiratory symptoms such as cough, breathlessness, and sputum production occur secondary to marijuana use (e.g., Ribeiro & Ind, 2018), although the evidence does not generally indicate that marijuana smoking alone causes pulmonary disease (e.g., Tan & Sin, 2018; Tashkin, 2018). However, smoking both marijuana and tobacco causes an additive effect, creating increased respiratory symptoms as well as a higher risk of chronic pulmonary disease (Tan et al., 2009). Smoking crack cocaine and the inhalation of cocaine or heroin can result in decreased pulmonary functioning, significant exacerbations of symptoms, and hospitalizations in asthma patients (e.g., Self, Shah, March, & Sands, 2017).

Smoking cessation is the only known intervention that can decrease the rate of lung function decline and the progression of pulmonary disease (Jiménez-Ruiz et al., 2015). Other treatments for chronic respiratory diseases (e.g., bronchodilators, inhaled corticosteroids) can help manage symptoms but do not stop disease progression. Smoking cessation results in improvements in the symptoms, but it will not return people to the lung function of those who have never smoked unless they quit early (i.e., before age 30; Kohansal et al., 2009).

ASSESSMENT AND BRIEF INTERVENTIONS AT DOCTOR VISITS

Because of the strong association between tobacco smoking and respiratory illness, clinical practice guidelines encourage medical providers to assess tobacco use in their patients and then to intervene to promote cessation if warranted (e.g., Clinical Practice Guideline Treating Tobacco Use and Dependence 2008 Update Panel, Liaisons, and Staff [CPG, 2008]). Known as the 5As model, medical professionals are encouraged to (a) *Ask* patients about tobacco use at each visit; (b) *Advise* patients to quit smoking; (c) *Assess* the patient's willingness to quit smoking; (d) *Assist* the patient with plans to quit, prescribe medication, and provide support; and (e) *Arrange* follow-up to monitor the patient's progress and provide additional intervention as needed. Several documents (e.g., CPG, 2008; Galvin, 2016) provide more detail on specific implementation strategies for each of the steps in the model. Some variation of this model is used by many primary care and pulmonary physicians, and research has demonstrated that abstinence is improved in those patients who receive the *Assist* and *Arrange* follow-up steps, rather than only the *Assessment* steps (Park et al., 2015; Quinn et al., 2009). This model is also useful to physicians for triage, to determine which patients will benefit from more in-depth intervention from a psychologist or other clinician who is trained in more extensive smoking cessation interventions.

SMOKING CESSATION INTERVENTIONS

Smokers average six to seven attempts to quit before successfully quitting (e.g., Agrawal & Britton, 2017). People who attempt to stop smoking typically experience withdrawal symptoms, including anxiety, cravings, irritability and mood changes, decreased concentration, stomach cramps, headache, insomnia, increased appetite, and tingling extremities. These symptoms can last up to a few weeks. There is some evidence that it is harder for patients with chronic lung disease to quit than for healthy people because they have greater dependence on nicotine (Jiménez-Ruiz et al., 2015; Perret, Boneveski, McDonald, & Abramson, 2016), slower decline of withdrawal symptoms and cravings (McLeish, Farris, Johnson, Bernstein, & Zvolensky, 2016), concern that smoking cessation may not make a difference (Alexis-Garsee, Gilbert, Burton, & van den Akker, 2018), and more depression than smokers without chronic lung disease (Jiménez-Ruiz et al., 2015). Smoking cessation interventions include nicotine replacement, pharmacotherapy, and psychological treatments. The overall goals of these interventions are to decrease withdrawal symptoms and cravings and to provide the individual with skills to avoid smoking.

Nicotine Replacement Therapy

There are many options for nicotine replacement therapy (NRT), including patches, gum, lozenges, microtabs, nasal or mouth spray, and inhalers; some NRT treatments are available over the counter, whereas others require a prescription. Foggo (2017) and WebMD (https://www.webmd.com/smoking-cessation/nicotine-replacement-therapy#1-2) provide more detail about each of these options.

NRT delivers nicotine to the individual at lower doses than smoking. The goals of NRT treatment are to wean people off the nicotine while managing withdrawal symptoms and cravings, and to do this without them inhaling the harmful toxins associated with cigarette smoking. However, NRT does not help people with the emotional and behavioral components of smoking, which is why a combination of NRT and counseling is often recommended (e.g., Tashkin, 2015). NRT is safe for most people; the most common side effects are skin or mouth irritation (depending on where the NRT is delivered; Hartmann-Boyce, Chepkin, Ye, Bullen, & Lancaster, 2018). Patients should be aware that they should not smoke cigarettes while using NRT because they could overdose on nicotine.

A Cochrane review of NRT for smoking cessation (Hartmann-Boyce et al., 2018) reported that its use increased the rate of quitting by 50% to 60%, with or without additional counseling. Physicians considering NRT for their patients will need to consider the best method of delivery, the dose and duration, and the usefulness of other therapies (e.g., counseling, bupropion) in combination with NRT. CPG (2008) and Tashkin (2015) provide information on decision making and dosing suggestions.

Electronic cigarettes (e-cigs) deliver a vapor that contains nicotine for inhalation. Smoking e-cigs (typically referred to as *vaping*) has been promoted as a method to help individuals decrease their nicotine intake while avoiding the other toxins associated with smoking traditional cigarettes.

These products may contain THC (tetrahydrocannabinol, the psychoactive ingredient in marijuana), other additives, and flavors that make them attractive to many. Initial research indicated that e-cigs enabled people to quit smoking with only a few side effects (Hartmann-Boyce et al., 2016). Recently, however, there have been many reported cases of lung injury and death in adolescents and adults due to the use of e-cigs. Vaping is popular and unregulated, and this has become a public health crisis. The CDC website (2019c) contains current information on the effects of e-cigs and is updated regularly. For now, patients should be strongly encouraged to use other methods for smoking cessation.

Pharmacotherapy

Several oral medications decrease cravings and withdrawal symptoms, including nortriptyline, clonidine, bupropion, and varenicline. GOLD (2018) reported that bupropion, varenicline, and nortriptyline increased long-term rates of quitting, but the rates are increased further if these medications are used in the context of a larger intervention program. Varenicline, in combination with cognitive behavior therapy or other support, demonstrated good abstinence results in smokers with COPD, asthma, and pneumonia (Hernández Zenteno et al., 2018; Politis, Ioannidis, Gourgoulianis, Daniil, & Hatzoglou, 2018). A review by Tashkin (2015) concluded that the effects of pharmacotherapy and NRT are improved when combined with even brief counseling. The most commonly used oral medications are bupropion and varenicline (discussed below).

Bupropion (Zyban), an antidepressant, is usually started 1 to 2 weeks prior to the quit date, then taken for at least 8 weeks (Foggo, 2017). It decreases cravings and withdrawal symptoms. One of the most serious potential side effects of bupropion is seizures, making it inappropriate for some patients (Agrawal & Britton, 2017).

Varenicline (Champix, Chantix) works by decreasing nicotine withdrawal symptoms and reducing the reward from nicotine (Foggo, 2017). As with bupropion, it is started prior to cessation. Varenicline is associated with several adverse side effects, including depression and suicidal ideation (Agrawal & Britton, 2017), so these need to be monitored.

Psychological Interventions

Traditional smoking cessation programs are effective with pulmonary patients (e.g., GOLD, 2018; Gratziou et al., 2014). Manualized treatments for group and individual intervention are available; one good option is the Primary

Care and Tobacco Cessation Handbook developed by the U.S. Department of Veterans Affairs (located at https://www.mentalhealth.va.gov/quit-tobacco/docs/IB_10-565-Primary-Care-Smoking-Handbook-PROVIDERS-508.pdf). This manual is focused on brief interventions for use in a primary care setting, but it provides a wealth of useful information, including educational material and scripts for talking with patients about cessation. McEwen, Hajek, McRobbie, and West (2006) provide additional examples of assessment and intervention strategies.

In many cases, psychologists will want to use an intervention program that incorporates issues specific to lung disease and is also tailored to the individual patient; specific smoking interventions are described below. Some research has demonstrated that psychological interventions in combination with NRT, e-cigarettes, or medication are most effective (e.g., Rigotti, 2013; Tashkin, 2015; van Eerd, van der Meer, van Schayck, & Kotz, 2016). Exhibit 8.1 is a useful handout for patients that can be used in conjunction with the change strategies described later.

Beyond the focus on smoking cessation, the psychological intervention may also target feelings of guilt or shame experienced by the patient. That is, many patients with COPD experience guilt because of the self-inflicted nature of the disease if they have smoked (see Lindqvist & Hallberg, 2010). For example, "It's just my own fault. If I hadn't been stupid enough to smoke, or had quit sooner, I would have been much better . . . there's no one [else] to blame" (Bragadottir, Halldorsdottir, Ingadottir, & Jonsdottir, 2018, p. 60). These negative feelings can make the quit process more difficult. However, as the patient experiences some success with quitting, he will often feel good about making healthier choices. Although current smoking cessation does not erase the effects of the poor choices in the past, it is what can be done now to take the best path forward.

Assessment and Education

To develop an appropriate smoking cessation treatment plan, it will be necessary to obtain information on the patient's smoking patterns, understand the reasons for smoking, past quit attempts, and other information relative to her smoking behavior. Education can be provided about effects of smoking, potential withdrawal symptoms, and treatments available to promote cessation.

Readiness to Change and Motivational Interviewing. The best interventions have little effect if the patient is not motivated to quit smoking. Therefore, it is important to assess the patient's readiness to quit initially and then

EXHIBIT 8.1. Tobacco Cessation

How to Change?

To effectively change your tobacco use, consider all of the factors that contribute to using tobacco. It can be helpful to group these factors into three main categories: physical factors, habits, and psychological (i.e., your thoughts and emotions).

Physically, nicotine is the most addictive substance on the planet. Your medical provider will tell you whether it is appropriate for you to use nicotine replacement, such as the patch or gum. Some medications, like Zyban, can help decrease cravings for tobacco.

Behaviorally, you will need to change your habits and the situations that you typically associate with tobacco. Undoubtedly, you will experience situations that cause you to crave tobacco, but you can learn skills that will help you choose alternatives to using tobacco.

Thoughts and emotions are some of the hardest aspects of tobacco use to change. Often individuals think that they need tobacco to get through a difficult situation. Changing these thoughts to cope with stress and negative emotions is an essential aspect of successful tobacco cessation.

Preparing to Quit

Your Quit Date

When is the last day and time that you are going to use tobacco?

Month   Day   Year   Time

Preparing Your Surroundings

What are the things that remind you to use tobacco? It is important to change your surroundings so that you won't be reminded about tobacco use as frequently. Before your quit date, consider the following:

- Don't buy tobacco in bulk (e.g., don't buy cartons).

- Find all of your hidden stashes of tobacco. Check in the couch, the glove compartment, in your drawers at home and at work—it is unwise to keep an emergency stash once you quit.

- Get rid of tobacco-related materials—things like ashtrays and lighters. You may need lighters for candles or fireplaces, but you likely don't need to carry lighters wherever you go.

- Prepare family and friends. Let them know that you are planning to quit and ask for their help. If you have friends and family who do use tobacco, ask them to avoid using tobacco around you.

- Choose a quit method. There are several ways to consider quitting, but one of the most important considerations is to avoid romanticizing your last tobacco use. If you remember your tobacco fondly, then you may be more likely to go back to tobacco use when you perceive that you need it. Here are some ways to avoid romanticizing your last use of tobacco:

  - *Nicotine fading.* Gradually decrease the amount of tobacco you are using. You can do this by decreasing how often you use your current tobacco, or you can switch to another brand of tobacco that has less nicotine.

(continues)

EXHIBIT 8.1. Tobacco Cessation (*Continued*)

- *Brand switching.* On the day that you are planning to quit, use a different brand of tobacco, preferably a brand that tastes stronger or significantly different from the brand that you use today. Rather than the pleasant sensation you associate with your current brand, you'll remember the more unpleasant taste of the new brand.

- *Aversive tobacco use.* The last time that you use tobacco, use a lot of it or use it quickly. Again, the idea is to have your last memory of tobacco be an unpleasant memory. So you might decide to smoke your last cigarette very rapidly, or use two or three times as much chewing tobacco as you normally would.

Using the Four As to Outsmart Tobacco Urges

Avoid. What are situations or places that you need to avoid over the next month?

1. _____
2. _____
3. _____

Alter. What situations will you need to change to help you be more successful?

1. _____
2. _____
3. _____

Alternatives. What can you put in your mouth or hands instead of using tobacco?

1. _____
2. _____
3. _____

Action. When you get an urge, what can you do to be active or busy?

1. _____
2. _____
3. _____

Note. Reprinted from *Integrated Behavioral Health in Primary Care: Step-by-Step Guidance for Assessment and Intervention* (2nd ed., pp. 89–90), by C. L. Hunter, J. L. Goodie, M. S. Oordt, and A. C. Dobmeyer, 2017, Washington, DC: American Psychological Association. Copyright 2017 by the American Psychological Association.

to intervene to improve readiness if necessary. Prochaska, DiClemente, and Norcross (1992) developed a model of the process of change that involves five stages: precontemplation, contemplation, preparation, action, and maintenance. Locating a patient within these stages can help a clinician to determine the intervention most likely to facilitate change in the patient. For example, individuals in the action stage are most ready to make changes in their behavior; interventions for those in earlier stages are most useful when they help people move toward readiness for action. Readiness to change can be assessed through an interview, but measures have also been developed to aid this process (see McConnaughy, DiClemente, Prochaska, & Velicer, 1989).

Motivational interviewing (MI) techniques are often used in the treatment of substance abuse, specifically to improve the patient's readiness for change when patients are uncertain or ambivalent about making a change that is in their best interest. The goal is to engage people in a discussion about change, especially the personal benefits of making the change. Because the benefits of abstinence from cigarette smoking are clear to most people, they can be asked to discuss the specific goal (cessation) and the specific changes in behavior that it will take to reach the goal. People are asked to review the importance of the change and discrepancies between the goal and their current behavior. (This is in contrast to the intervention the patient likely gets from his doctor, where he is typically told the risks of smoking, the benefits of quitting, and then told to quit. This often results in a response such as "Yeah, I know" and no motivation to change.) The end result is for the patient to articulate the goal, see that it is worthwhile to achieve, understand what needs to be done, and view the goal as reachable. Once patients are ready to change, smoking cessation interventions will be more successful. See Miller and Rollnick (2013) and Anstiss and Passmore (2012) for more detail and specific examples of MI techniques.

Education. Pulmonary patients are typically aware that smoking is "bad" for them, but they are often unaware of the impacts of smoking on respiratory disease (see the Respiratory Effects of Smoking Tobacco and Other Substances section earlier in this chapter). Patients need to understand information about their specific disease and smoking. For example, a patient with TB needs to know that smoking is associated with more frequent infections, whereas a patient with COPD needs to know that smoking is associated with decreased lung function, faster disease progression, and increased mortality.

Even though many patients have attempted to quit smoking in the past, they can often benefit from additional education on the process and experience. People can be educated about specific withdrawal symptoms that they may experience, how long these are likely to occur, and suggestions to manage them. They can be educated about triggers for smoking behavior, cravings, and ways to cope with them. Finally, people should be aware that these discomforts will decrease over time but that they may still experience some of them even years after they have successfully quit.

Patients should also be educated about treatments to help them quit and to abstain from tobacco, for example, NRT, psychological interventions, combination treatments, and weight control methods. They can be alerted to web-based information and interventions to aid their cessation efforts. All education should be provided in lay terms and with written information to reinforce the in-person education.

Reasons for Smoking and Past Failures to Quit. The psychologist will need to thoroughly evaluate the patient's smoking history. Current smoking frequency is important, as well as specific and detailed information on the situations in which the person smokes. Triggers for smoking and details about past quit attempts will also be needed.

Understanding an individual's reasons for smoking can help with cessation because these specific issues can be explicitly addressed in the treatment. Some of the more common reasons for smoking include habit, stress reduction, a shared social event, and smoking as part of the individual's identity. Events associated with these specific triggers are often associated with past failures to quit.

Many feel that smoking helps them to manage stress. However, in stressful situations, smoking is often paired with removing themselves from the situation to a quieter and calmer location where they can collect themselves and calm down. It may be these other components that are actually responsible for the stress reduction; most people have never considered that other aspects of the situation also promote stress reduction. If people attribute feeling emotionally better to smoking, rather than to other aspects of the situation, they are at risk for relapse if a difficult situation occurs in their lives (e.g., the familiar scenario in which a person smokes to relieve stress and successfully quits until he loses his job and then relapses). Other strategies to manage stress (e.g., relaxation, coping) can be included in the treatment program to decrease this risk.

Individuals may also find that they bond with others over situations that involve smoking (e.g., in bars or at other social events). Here, it is useful to consider how they can obtain the social benefits of those events without smoking, that is, they can develop plans to help them face those situations (and triggers) without smoking, or they can find ways to derive the social benefits in other contexts that do not involve smoking.

Some people feel smoking is part of their identity; reconsidering who they are and what aspects of themselves are most important can be useful. Others smoke only out of habit, and people can learn strategies to break the habit and replace it with other, more adaptive behaviors. Ultimately, knowing the role that smoking plays for the individual can enable the development of a treatment plan to address that specifically.

Self-Monitoring and Quit Date. Some patients will want to spend a few weeks decreasing cigarette smoking before quitting, whereas others will quickly set a full-stop date. In either case, individuals can benefit from monitoring their smoking behavior, cravings, and triggers. Self-monitoring (either on paper or electronically) will keep their attention on the behavior, may enable them to decrease tobacco use prior to quitting completely, and will also provide valuable information about their vulnerabilities, which can then be targeted in treatment.

Cognitive and Behavioral Interventions

People need to change behaviors to help them quit and remain abstinent from smoking. One strategy is to change patterns of behavior that involve smoking; for example, one woman would always smoke her first cigarette in the morning prior to getting out of bed and beginning her day. Her behavioral plans to address this habit included having no cigarettes in the house; getting immediately out of bed, brushing her teeth, and getting on with her day; and managing cravings by calling her sister or taking a walk. Some people need to keep their hands and mouth busy and could, as an alternative, hold a pen or chew a straw temporarily.

Individuals also need to learn that events that were once associated with smoking are no longer associated with smoking; thus, she no longer has a cigarette after dinner with a cup of coffee, but the individual can have coffee alone, pair it with something else, or skip it altogether. She also needs to remind herself that any of these options is fine, that she will get used to this, and that the benefits of working on this will be worth it in the long term.

Goal setting with appropriate reinforcement can help people to make behavioral changes, either to cut back initially or to maintain abstinence. They should select appropriate reinforcers for the short term (e.g., attend a movie or buy a book after four days of abstinence) as well as larger rewards (e.g., buy a new phone or take a weekend vacation) after 6 or 12 months of abstinence.

Cognitive strategies can also help with smoking cessation. When people experience cravings, they can often work their way through them successfully, using cognitions such as "this will get easier," "it will all be worth it when I can breathe better," or "I can handle this." Keeping in mind the short-term relief from the craving versus the longer term medical problems (e.g., more difficulty breathing, physical limitations, disability) can often help them manage the craving. Individuals may also need to reconceptualize their identity; for example, rather than thinking of themselves as individuals who fail at smoking cessation, they should now think of themselves as nonsmokers (because this attempt is different from the others and is more likely to be successful).

Relapse prevention (RP) is "a cognitive-behavioral approach that combines behavioral skills training procedures with cognitive intervention techniques to assist persons in maintaining desired behavioral changes" (Douaihy, Stowell, Park, & Daley, 2007, p. 38). One aspect of RP is to have people develop plans to avoid a lapse (smoking after quitting) or a relapse (beginning to smoke regularly again). Initially, individuals develop a list of high-risk situations likely to elicit cravings or wishes to smoke (e.g., first thing in the morning, after a meal, at a party). The clinician then helps the patient to develop plans to manage these situations without smoking, using coping strategies, problem-solving skills, and cognitive restructuring. Experiences of success in these situations will increase the person's confidence in her or his ability to cope with these situations in the future, making it more likely that he or she can maintain abstinence. (Douaihy et al., 2007, and Witkiewitz & Marlatt, 2007, provide specific examples of RP techniques.)

If a lapse does occur, it is important to address that situation to ensure that the person does not revert to the old behavior (relapse). Witkiewitz and Marlatt (2007) provide a list of cognitive and behavioral steps to take if a lapse occurs to avoid it becoming a relapse. Specifically, individuals need to attend to what has happened but not overreact to it. They should remember their successes and learn what they can from the mistake so they can avoid another one. They should make plans to help themselves at the moment they are at risk. Finally, people should deal with the abstinence violation effect (the feeling that once they have made a mistake, they might as well give up). Case 8.1 is an example of a patient's making plans to quit and managing a lapse.

Social Support

Any and all support can be helpful to patients as they work to quit smoking and remain abstinent. Support from professionals can be demonstrated through encouragement, attention to the patients' concerns and struggles, reinforcing successes, and helping them to develop confidence (CPG, 2008, provides specific suggestions). Some patients will find group treatments for smoking cessation helpful because social support is built into the program. Additional online and web-based resources can provide support and additional tips for smoking cessation.

CASE 8.1

SMOKING CESSATION

Mr. L was a 50-year-old man recently diagnosed with COPD. He had smoked for 25 years at a moderate level. He understood the need to stop smoking, but he had tried several times in the past without long-term success. The patient's internist prescribed bupropion to aid the patient's quit efforts and referred him for psychological intervention.

As the patient had made quit attempts before, he was aware of potential withdrawal symptoms, the need to break old patterns, and the benefits of rewarding himself for successes. He already had good plans to address those issues. He noted that he had done fairly well with quitting in the past, but he tended to begin smoking again when attending social situations in which other people smoked. The initial intervention, then, was to help the patient plan for the social situations in which he was at risk. He noted that Sunday barbecues with family were particularly difficult for him. He felt he was at most risk when drinking beer and helping his brother grill dinner. The patient was able to articulate specific events that make it more likely that he will be tempted to smoke (his brother lighting a cigarette, having more than one beer, spending a lot of time with the cooking). He considered some initial actions that he could take, such as taking kitchen (rather than grill) duty, waiting to have a beer until after the dinner was cooked, drinking a beverage with a straw so that he had something in his mouth, and asking his brother to not offer him a cigarette. He was also able to generate coping strategies to manage cravings/temptations when they did occur. These included cognitions about the benefits of not smoking, the fact that quitting would get easier over time, and that he has the ability to quit successfully. If it looked like he was close to smoking, he could simply walk away, placing himself in a different situation until he felt he had regained control.

At his next session, the Monday after the barbecue, he reported that "it didn't go well." He reported smoking one cigarette when grilling with his brother, in spite of following all of his plans. He initially felt good that he had only one, but he quickly became concerned that this would be as unsuccessful as his other quit attempts. He continued to berate himself for the lapse and ultimately smoked another cigarette later in the evening.

The intervention was to help the patient to conceptualize this as a mistake on his path to success, rather than another failure. He was able to generate cognitions consistent with this idea (e.g., "One mistake will not blow the whole plan") and also some that reminded him of his successes

(continues)

CASE 8.1
SMOKING CESSATION (*Continued*)

(e.g., "I have been doing pretty well overall"). He was reminded that this is not like all his other quit attempts because he has additional motivation, resources, and tools available to help him this time. He was encouraged to use these two lapses as learning experiences. The patient knew that he smoked in the evening because he was upset about the initial lapse earlier in the day. He felt that the cognitions just discussed combined with some distraction techniques would enable him to manage that upset if it occurred again. He was stumped, though, about what triggered the initial lapse. He felt he was not upset at the barbecue; he was happy and was not experiencing any significant cravings at the time. After some discussion he decided that smoking in that situation was a strong habit and that it was a bonding experience with his brother. He decided that he would not be able to grill with his brother for now, and he would do other chores in the house at grilling time. He felt he had ample other opportunities to bond with his brother so this would not be a hardship.

Mr. L's plan for the next barbecue involved preparing himself with reminders of the adaptive cognitions he had generated. He planned to avoid grilling with his brother in the near future. He felt that if these plans did not work, he would stop attending the weekly barbecues. This was acknowledged as a possible option in the short term, but it was not a good long-term strategy because he would lose valuable social contact and would also not improve his skills to manage situations such as these.

Support from significant people in the patient's life is often difficult to obtain even though this is the most immediately relevant support for the patient; family and friends may even be actively nonsupportive. Many people have been nagged to quit smoking for years, an experience usually perceived as demeaning and not helpful. Patients may be able to educate their significant others about what behaviors they would perceive as helpful, such as leaving the room if they smoke, avoiding social events where others smoke (at least initially), or saying no if the patient asks for a cigarette. Supportive others can also help the patient to see progress and to feel good about choices they have made.

Unfortunately, some people in the patient's life may actively encourage them to smoke. This can occur when others express beliefs that the individual will be unable to quit successfully ("Why bother, you didn't stick to it last time"), actively disregard the patient's struggles (offering a cigarette), or simply forget that the patient is working to quit. The patient may be able to communicate to the family member what would be more helpful, and at times the psychologist may meet with both parties to provide education and plans to improve support.

To conclude, a word about hypnosis: Long used as a treatment for smoking cessation, hypnosis is popular with some patients because it takes less time and effort than most psychological interventions. However, the evidence on its usefulness as a treatment for smoking cessation is mixed (e.g., Green & Lynn, 2019; Shirley, 2006), and it is most likely to be useful when used as part of a comprehensive program for smoking cessation. Green and Lynn (2019) provided details of an intervention for smoking cessation that combines hypnosis with cognitive behavior therapy and mindfulness.

9 FAMILY CHALLENGES AND SOCIAL SUPPORT

Family members of a patient with chronic respiratory disease play a variety of roles. At the initial psychological evaluation, they can be an important source of collateral information that can help the psychologist develop an appropriate treatment plan (see Chapter 4). Toward the end of a patient's life, family members may need to make decisions about the patient's medical care and treatment during his final days (see Chapter 10). Throughout the process, family members have the opportunity to provide support to the patient and can play an important part in the patient's successful management of her disease. Family members may experience significant impacts of the patient's disease as roles and family relationships change.

FAMILY AND CAREGIVER BURDEN

The diagnosis of any serious illness for a family member can be a source of stress for the family. Some respiratory diseases (e.g., chronic obstructive pulmonary disease [COPD]) may not be diagnosed until they have progressed to a significant level; others have been diagnosed early in life (e.g., cystic

http://dx.doi.org/10.1037/0000189-010
Psychological Treatment of Patients With Chronic Respiratory Disease, by S. M. Labott

fibrosis [CF]). Dealing with the disease may involve fears among multiple or all family members about losing the family member, changes in roles within the family, and limitations on the family's activities.

One recent study described the experiences of patients and family members as they went through the process of coming to terms with COPD (Bragadottir, Halldorsdottir, Ingadottir, & Jonsdottir, 2018). Others have reported on the experiences of couples (Ek, Ternestedt, Andershed, & Sahlberg-Blom, 2011) and families (Gabriel, Figueiredo, Jácome, Cruz, & Marques, 2014) when one family member has severe COPD. The challenges (summarized below) that emerged from these three studies are similar and speak to concerns about (a) dealing with uncertainty, (b) changes in the relationship, (c) challenges to understanding and communication, and (d) increased responsibilities for the healthy partner. Note that many aspects of family life can be affected by chronic respiratory disease.

Living with uncertainty was demonstrated in the spouse's (and also the patient's) fears that something bad could happen at any time. Some couples had experienced the quick development of symptoms that had led to medical emergencies. One patient had become unconscious in the past; his spouse said,

> I do get scared when he gets those coughing fits. He can't catch his breath at all, and then there's the phlegm . . . it sounds horrible. I usually try to shake some life into him, and he responds after a while. If he's sitting out there, if he starts while I'm in the kitchen, I can hear how far gone he is [unconscious]. (Ek et al., 2011, p. 192)

Patients and spouses acknowledged their hopes that things would improve with more intense treatment (e.g., oxygen), but they also realized that a treatment such as this was another sign of the severity of the COPD and the fact that death could occur at any time.

Partners also reported changes in the relationship. One aspect of this was intimacy; as sexual activity decreased, the relationship was more about companionship. If the spouse with COPD also required help with bathing, toileting, and other personal activities, both spouses needed to adjust to a different type of intimacy and role changes. The larger family's social life also changed, resulting in a reduction in social contacts and fewer social activities outside of the home.

Problems with understanding and communication occurred frequently. In some cases, spouses had difficulty slowing their pace to accommodate the partner who became breathless when walking, and it was often not discussed. Conversation was also affected by shortness of breath, and silence from a breathless partner was at times misunderstood as anger, leading to further stress in the relationship. The healthy spouse sometimes blamed the partner with COPD for the development of the illness, and patients also often blamed themselves.

The healthy partner generally had to take on additional responsibilities, such as tasks around the house, picking up medications, and taking the patient with COPD to medical appointments. Healthy partners reported feeling alone and that they had little support from family and medical professionals. Families also noted new financial problems due to expensive treatments and decreased income if the spouse with COPD could no longer work.

These concerns highlight the stressful and emotional issues that partners and family members of chronic pulmonary patients may face daily and for a long period of time. The salience of these issues is likely to depend on the severity of the pulmonary disease and the premorbid health of the relationship.

Anxiety and depression occur commonly in family caregivers of chronic respiratory disease patients; anxiety has been reported in 46% to 63%, depression in 23% to 40%, and 27% of caregivers or partners report both (Jácome, Figueiredo, Gabriel, Cruz, & Marques, 2014; Mi et al., 2017; Papaioannou et al., 2014). Depression and anxiety in the partner are correlated with depression and anxiety in the patient (Mi et al., 2017). Partner depression is also associated with the patient's disease severity (Papaioannou et al., 2014).

Dyadic coping (the way partners deal with stress) is also associated with the burden of COPD. That is, low levels of negative (e.g., hostile provision of help) and high levels of positive (supportive assistance) dyadic coping are associated with better quality of life and less distress in couples with COPD (Meier, Bodenmann, Moergeli, & Jenewein, 2011). If patients reported unbalanced support in the relationship, that is, high support *from* their partner but low provision of support *to* their partner, both partners reported poorer quality of life (Meier et al., 2012). Further, when compared with healthy couples, couples with COPD also reported more negative and unbalanced coping overall.

Disease severity seems also to affect the coping strategies used by caregivers and caregiver burden (Figueiredo, Gabriel, Jácome, & Marques, 2014). Three types of coping were studied, using the Carers' Assessment of Managing Index (Brito, 2002): (a) problem-solving strategies (e.g., planning, seeking information, getting help), (b) emotional–cognitive (e.g., remembering good times, taking it one day at a time), and (c) dealing with the stress consequences (e.g., letting off steam, having a good cry). These researchers reported that caregivers of people with early COPD used fewer problem-solving and emotional–cognitive strategies than caregivers of patients with advanced COPD. Dealing with the stress consequences was the least used by both groups. Problem-solving was perceived as the most useful coping in caregivers of both the early and advanced groups, and it was associated with physical health in the caregivers of patients with advanced COPD. Others have reported that caregivers of people with advanced COPD report more depression, poorer mental health, and greater burden (Figueiredo, Gabriel, Jácome, Cruz, & Marques, 2014).

At times, it is most useful to include family members in some of the patient's psychological treatment, especially when providing information or when teaching coping or relaxation strategies that can benefit both. The patient and family member can then support each other as they learn to manage the stressors associated with respiratory disease. However, in most cases, a family member should be referred for his or her own psychological treatment, so that both parties have individual attention and intervention to address their concerns.

SOCIAL SUPPORT

Social support has been defined in many ways but generally refers to the resources provided by others to help an individual cope with stress or to function generally. Social support is often conceptualized as involving two components:

- *Instrumental support* includes practical and physical help to accomplish activities, for example, providing transportation to an appointment, ordering medications and organizing them, or doing laundry and other chores.

- *Emotional support* involves such behaviors as providing encouragement, understanding, and helping with motivation.

Social support is often assessed by counting the number of supportive people in a person's life, or with questionnaires that ask people to rate support from others, given a list of specific behaviors that reflect instrumental and emotional support. Social relationships and support have been associated with improved mental and physical health, adherence, and survival (e.g., DiMatteo, 2004a; Holt-Lunstad, 2018).

A distinction has been made between *perceived* and *received* support. Perceived support is the individual's assessment of support that is available to him; received support is a more objective rating of the support that has actually been provided to the individual. Perceived support has been consistently related to mental health and increased survival, but the findings for received support are less consistent and seem to be influenced by other variables (see Knoll, Scholz, & Ditzen, 2019, for a review). Some specific behaviors may be intended as supportive by a family member but may not be perceived as such by the recipient, such as when a family member is "too helpful" and does not allow a patient to engage in behaviors she is able to do. Alternately, a supportive behavior may not be experienced as such if the spouse who delivers it is perceived as angry or disinterested.

In the initial stages, others may be unaware that a person has a chronic respiratory disease, and social support may not be forthcoming. Patients may struggle with the issue of who to tell about the disease. If they smoked, they may feel stigmatized and guilty about their role in the development of the disease. They may be unwilling to seek social support because they feel they do not deserve it, and some significant others may be more willing to punish them than to provide support.

As the disease progresses, people are at risk of losing social relationships and the support that derives from them. If others are unaware of the disease, they may begin to avoid a patient with symptoms (especially cough) because they fear being exposed to an infectious illness that they might catch. Additionally, if pulmonary patients curtail certain social activities because they involve too much exertion, the social relationships associated with those activities may suffer. It may take effort to find ways that the patient can attend these events while avoiding exertion or to find new activities through which the patient can connect with family and friends. Patients may also need to develop new relationships that are associated with more manageable physical activities, for example, with new friends from pulmonary rehabilitation.

Family support has been associated with improved mental health and lower levels of anxiety and depression in those with asthma (Smyth, Zawadzki, Santuzzi, & Filipkowski, 2014), silicosis (Han et al., 2014), COPD (Barton, Effing, & Cafarella, 2015; Tselebis et al., 2013), and CF (Flewelling, Sellers, Sawicki, Robinson, & Dill, 2019). Unsupportive families are associated with emotional distress, dyspnea, and poorer quality of life (Holm, Bowler, Make, & Wamboldt, 2009; Holm, LaChance, Bowler, Make, & Wamboldt, 2010). Social support is associated with more physical activity in COPD (Chen, Fan, Belza, Pike, & Nguyen, 2017) and fewer physical symptoms and better functioning in CF (Flewelling et al., 2019). Social support can be helpful to patients as they attempt to quit smoking (see Chapter 8). In contrast, unsupportive family relationships are associated with emotional distress, which is associated with smoking (Holm et al., 2010).

FACILITATING FAMILY SUPPORT

Many patients are fortunate enough to have partners and families who want to do their best to support the patient. In these cases, providing information to the family (about the disease and the patient's needs) can help family members to determine their role in supporting the patient. The psychologist can meet with family members, providing them with information and giving them handouts, or directing them to a reputable website such as WebMD (http://webmd.com) or the Mayo Clinic (http://mayoclinic.org), so that they can become educated about the disease and symptoms. Family members can be helped to develop appropriate expectations for their family member and can develop an understanding about his or her specific needs. The patient can also participate by articulating specifically what he or she needs and wants; these requests can then be discussed openly with the family. Patients often need to be reminded that families have no chance of meeting their needs if they do not know what the needs are.

Common requests of respiratory patients are consistent with the relationship challenges noted above. That is, pulmonary patients often want help with instrumental activities, such as having a family member keep a calendar of appointments, manage medications, or provide help with chest physiotherapy or transportation to appointments. They also request demonstrations of understanding, such as being dropped off at the door, rather than walking a long distance from where the car is parked, or asking that family members remember that walking can be difficult and not tell them to "hurry up." Patients often desire better communication and emotional support, evidenced by efforts to keep them involved in family matters even if they cannot do the physical activities they used to, helping them to maintain motivation for rehab and other aspects of the medical regimen, and collaborating to distinguish helping from nagging. Patients may wish that spouses also quit smoking in support of the patient's efforts, or they may want to problem solve ways they can remain connected to people while engaging in less physical activity. Although they provide information about what a patient may perceive as supportive, all of these behaviors need to be tailored to the needs of a specific patient on the basis of her or his physical, cognitive, and emotional status.

Although patients will commonly say that their kids or other family members are "too busy" to help, that is often not the case if the family is educated about the patient's needs. However, there are cases in which a family member is unable (e.g., because of their own physical limitations) or unwilling to deliver what is required to support the patient and his care. In these situations, family members should not be given significant responsibilities. Patients are usually quite aware if a family member has a history of irresponsible behavior. One patient with COPD developed pneumonia and spent several weeks in the hospital and then in an inpatient rehabilitation program. Her son was enlisted to manage her finances while she was in the hospital and to coordinate her medical appointments and manage her medications when she was discharged back home. It took a few weeks for the patient's medical providers to realize that the son was not giving the patient her medications as prescribed, that he had allowed her to run out of some of them, and that he was not getting her to her medical appointments consistently. Further, he had not paid her utility bills but had run up her credit card bill on things that he wanted for himself. Changes were then made, and the patient received outside services to help her with her medications and appointments. She returned to paying her own bills, but it took her a long time (financially and emotionally) to recover from this.

Fortunately, most families do better. Case 9.1 presents a patient who was beginning to need help at home. Her grown children had the best intentions and were good at problem-solving, but they also had concerns and financial constraints that affected their ability to help. Note that the psychological interventions were not focused on their own personal issues but were geared to help them manage their concerns as they served as caregivers for their mother.

CASE 9.1

CHRONIC OBSTRUCTIVE PULMONARY DISEASE AND FAMILY SUPPORT

Mrs. X is a 76-year-old Caucasian woman, referred by her pulmonologist with concerns about her ability to live alone. She recently forgot to fill one of her medications and was not aware of the problem until she had to be admitted to the hospital with a COPD exacerbation. She was discharged 3 days ago. Mrs. X arrived for her appointment with her adult son. She was initially interviewed alone.

(continues)

CASE 9.1

CHRONIC OBSTRUCTIVE PULMONARY DISEASE AND FAMILY SUPPORT *(Continued)*

She reports that she has been widowed for the past 7 years and lives alone. She has a daughter and a son. She completed college and is a retired bookkeeper.

Mrs. X reports multiple medical problems, including coronary artery disease, COPD, hypertension, and hypercholesterolemia. She takes a variety of medications at several times throughout the day and uses a nebulizer. She has no physical impairments except shortness of breath with moderate exertion.

She has frequent medical appointments and reports that much of her time is spent attending to her medical issues. She has a good understanding of what her medical regimen involves and the rationale for each aspect of it. She reports good compliance with all aspects of her medical regimen but acknowledges that she recently forgot to refill one of her prescriptions. She feels that trying to follow all the medical recommendations and take prescriptions on time is causing her significant stress recently. She worries that she will do something wrong and that her health will deteriorate as a result. She reports no other problems with living home alone except that she left the stove on once recently. Her neighbor's daughter comes once weekly to do her laundry and to help with household chores.

Mrs. X reported no previous inpatient or outpatient psychological treatment, no psychotropic medications, no suicide attempts, and no family history of psychological problems. She reports an episode of depression after her husband died, but she did not seek treatment and it resolved on its own in about 8 months.

Mrs. X denied current feelings of depression, hopelessness, helplessness, suicidal ideation, sleep or appetite problems, anxiety, and hallucinations. She does report some worry about managing her medications and about a grandson who has a drug problem. She acknowledges some concerns about her memory recently.

On a mental status exam, Mrs. X was alert and oriented × 4. Her registration, attention, and long-term memory were all intact. Her short-term memory was moderately impaired (1/3 at 5 min), and her judgment was intact. Her speech was normal in rate and rhythm, and her mood was good. She was able to accurately follow a three-stage command.

The clinician explained and discussed the following feedback with Mrs. X: (a) no significant psychological history or current symptoms; (b) mental status OK except for short-term memory; (c) she has a good understanding of medical issues and the regimen, but she is beginning to have memory

CASE 9.1
CHRONIC OBSTRUCTIVE PULMONARY DISEASE AND FAMILY SUPPORT (*Continued*)

problems likely to affect adherence and perhaps her ability to live independently. The clinician also discussed options to address this concern, for example, move to an assisted living facility or enlist additional help at home. She agreed with this assessment and the recommendations, and she requested that her son be invited in to discuss this feedback further.

The feedback was reviewed with her son, and he agreed with the conclusions and recommendations. The compliance and safety concerns were also reviewed. Mrs. X's son had concerns about the patient remaining at home and preferred that she go to some kind of a facility, perhaps a nursing home, where she would be looked after and the family would not need to worry. Mrs. X argued that she was generally fine but just needed a little help. A meeting was scheduled for the next week with the patient, her son, and her daughter. In the meantime, the patient's granddaughter (who was home from college briefly) would move in with her and help out.

The following week, the son again argued for putting her into a nursing home. The daughter was pushing for assisted living because it would allow her mother more independence. The patient simply wanted to stay home and felt she would be alright with minimal help; she began to cry because she felt that her children wanted to put her into a facility when she did not yet need or want that.

The son reported being concerned about being responsible for his mother and her health. He had little understanding of COPD, her symptoms, and how to manage them. They were given some basic information and referred to the WebMD website for more. Mrs. X was able to convince her son that she was able to handle the symptoms of her disease and also her activities of daily living, such as bathing and feeding. The son seemed more comfortable if he didn't need to be responsible for any of those activities. Both of the patient's children were somewhat overwhelmed at the time and effort it might take to keep their mother at home safely. However, although hesitant, the son and daughter ultimately agreed for a trial of her staying at home to see how it would go.

The specific needs of the patient were reviewed. Because she had been independent at home and doing well for the most part, she did not need continual supervision. However, she did need help with her medication and meals as well as transportation to appointments. Options to manage each of these issues were discussed, and the family agreed to continue the discussion and return with plans to address these at the next visit, scheduled for 4 days later.

(continues)

CASE 9.1

CHRONIC OBSTRUCTIVE PULMONARY DISEASE AND FAMILY SUPPORT (*Continued*)

The family had made some decisions by the next appointment and had developed a comprehensive plan of what they would do to help their mother stay in her home:

1. Her son had begun to manage her medications and organized them in a pill box for her. He also had developed an alarm system using her phone so that an alarm would sound when it was time for her to take medication or use the nebulizer, and she had a list to refer to that indicated what she did at what times of day. The patient had been organizing her treatments herself until recently, and this provided her with additional reminders to keep her adherent. Mrs. X felt less stressed with these plans in place.

2. The patient's daughter planned to stop by her mother's house several times weekly to cook dinner for her, and, on days the daughter was not there, Mrs. X would get carryout from a restaurant down the block. She went grocery shopping with her neighbor weekly and planned to continue to do so. She agreed that she would not use the stove if she was home alone.

3. Mrs. X's son agreed to take her to medical appointments.

4. Her daughter and son each committed to spending two nights per week overnight at the patient's house.

5. They bought their mother a medical alert bracelet in case she needed help when they were away (and she was getting used to wearing it). Two of the patient's neighbors had also agreed to help in an emergency, and their phone numbers were posted by the telephone.

The family seemed mildly overwhelmed by all the changes and by the responsibility they were taking on, but they were resistant to bringing in other help, largely because of financial concerns. They now felt strongly that they needed to be responsible for all these tasks, and they felt they could do so successfully. They were educated about the stressors that can be associated with caregiving and about the importance of caring for themselves and their own families as well. They were also reminded to allow their mother as much independence as was safe for her.

The family returned after a month. At this point, the patient was stable medically, cognitively, and emotionally. She was taking her medications properly, was not using the stove when alone, and she wore her medical alert bracelet. She had been unable to schedule all of her medical appointments when her son was off work, so she missed two appointments.

CASE 9.1

CHRONIC OBSTRUCTIVE PULMONARY DISEASE AND FAMILY SUPPORT (*Continued*)

The family agreed to look into a transport service that could take her to appointments when he was working. They had originally rejected that idea because they were concerned about the expense, but the social worker had recently located a transport service that would be covered by the patient's insurance. After a few weeks, it had become clear that Mrs. X's daughter would be unable to do the cooking that she had planned at her mother's home, so she began to bring the patient leftovers from the meals that she made for her own family. The carry-outs from the nearby restaurant became too expensive so that plan was dropped. However, the daughter bringing leftovers from home was working out well for her own schedule, and Mrs. X was content with it. Her son had been unable to spend the overnights with his mother as planned because of overtime at work that interfered, and his sister was unable to spend additional time because she had adolescents at home who needed her attention.

Both children were now beginning to feel guilty about what they were unable to do, but the patient was doing well and was comfortable with these changes. Managing their emotions and frustrations in these new roles was discussed, as well as options to bring in additional help as needed. The family planned to return in another month.

In spite of good adherence to her medical regimen and getting regular meals, it was clear in another month that Mrs. X had begun to deteriorate physically and was having more respiratory distress. Her short-term memory was impaired at times, and she had again occasionally missed doses of medication. She had seen her pulmonologist and the management of her symptoms was maximized. Son and daughter now were unwilling to try to keep her in her home. Although Mrs. X was not happy about this, she was willing to accept a move to an assisted living facility (although not a nursing home). The family was now actively looking for a facility that would meet her needs and that she could afford. They were optimistic that they would find the right placement and would get her moved in the next few months. In the meantime, the patient was planning to live with her daughter and her family.

Mrs. X's children seemed to be managing this well and were sent to the waiting room. The patient denied significant anxiety or depression and seemed to be coping adequately with the changes in her life. She was educated about resources for psychological intervention after her move to the assisted living facility. The family was scheduled for another visit a month later, with the understanding that they could cancel if they no longer needed it.

10 END OF LIFE

Most patients with chronic lung disease do not receive specialized end-of-life (EOL) care. Although hospice care is focused on comfort, maximizing the patient's quality of life, and providing support for patients and families, only about 6% of patients with chronic obstructive pulmonary disease (COPD) die in hospice, in contrast to 34% who die in the hospital (Yaqoob, Al-Kindi, & Zein, 2017). Patients often do not access this care because they do not know they are dying. End-stage COPD patients feel they have more time and that they will "bounce back" as they have in the past (Lowey, Norton, Quinn, & Quill, 2013). Many have experienced a slow decline in their functioning over years, with occasional exacerbations and hospitalizations, and they may not realize that they are now close to death. They voice concerns that their health is deteriorating, and they understand that this could be life-threatening, but they do not understand that their disease is life-threatening *now*.

Similarly, physicians find it difficult to determine when a patient is in a terminal phase of the illness and, so, are less likely to refer respiratory patients to EOL care (Beernaert et al., 2013). As a result, many patients with end-stage lung disease remain at home, struggling with difficult symptoms (most commonly breathlessness, fatigue, pain, anxiety, and depression;

http://dx.doi.org/10.1037/0000189-011
Psychological Treatment of Patients With Chronic Respiratory Disease, by S. M. Labott

Solano, Gomes, & Higginson, 2006) and severe limitations. At some point they will likely have an acute exacerbation of symptoms and go to the hospital, where they die sometime later (Rajala et al., 2016).

DOCUMENTING END-OF-LIFE DECISIONS

Any person with a chronic and progressive lung disease should consider their wishes for EOL treatment, document these decisions, and share them with family members. The best time for patients to document their wishes is before they are actually facing the end of life. Patients can document their wishes and provide them to the physician at any time, and the doctor can place them into the medical record. In reality, however, many of these decisions are made within a few days of the patient's death (Rajala et al., 2016).

One of the best ways to address wishes for EOL care is through the use of advance directives. The Patient Self-Determination Act of 1990 (https://www.congress.gov/bill/101st-congress/house-bill/4449/text) requires that certain institutions (e.g., hospitals, nursing homes) offer patients the option of completing advance directives so that others will know their wishes for treatment and care if the patient is unable to articulate them. Patients can also designate someone as their power of attorney for health care who will make decisions on their behalf if they are unable to do so. The National Hospice and Palliative Care Organization (http://www.nhpco.org/advance-care-planning) provides information on advance directives and relevant forms for use in each state. Many patients find it useful to review the forms and then discuss them with their physician prior to formally completing them. A final copy should be given to medical providers and family.

Patients can also complete living wills—similar to an advance directive but more limited in scope—in which they document what measures they do or do not want at the end of their lives. One of the most common provisions of living wills involves a "do not resuscitate" (DNR) order. For pulmonary patients, of most relevance is a "do not intubate" (DNI) order. Many pulmonary patients are comfortable with intubation (being placed on a ventilator) if it is a temporary procedure to keep them alive while a medical problem is being resolved, but they are not willing to be intubated if it will be permanent and is simply a way to prolong a life that has no quality. Through a living will, patients can indicate their wishes about a variety of measures, such as intubation, nutrition, and hydration.

Some states also have documents called Physician Orders for Life-Sustaining Treatment (POLST; e.g., National POLST Paradigm, n.d.; Pope & Hexum, 2012). POLST is intended for people who could die within the next year and provides more specific directions regarding treatment than the general guidelines found in advance directives. Bomba, Kemp, and Black (2012) provide a copy of a POLST document and a case demonstrating how the use of POLST can improve the likelihood that a patient's wishes are followed.

Some states have death with dignity legislation for patients wishing assisted suicide. Although rules differ by state, in most cases a patient must have a terminal diagnosis, have decisional capacity, and one or two physicians need to document that. Some states require a psychological evaluation if the patient's ability to make her own decisions is in question. See the Compassion & Choices website (https://compassionandchoices.org/) for more information on death with dignity, advance directives, and other EOL issues.

WITHHOLDING AND TERMINATING TREATMENT

Most often, a patient's EOL medical decisions are handled at the moment the patient is facing a specific problem in the acute care setting. If it becomes clear to the patient's doctors that ongoing medical treatment is futile, they will begin discussions with the patient or family about the likely course for the patient with or without more treatment. Information is typically provided about DNR and DNI, as well as about withholding or withdrawing additional treatment such as antibiotics, nutrition, or hydration, and it will include a recommendation about the best course of action.

For a pulmonary patient whose treatment is futile and who requires mechanical ventilation to continue breathing, a decision may be made to remove the patient from the ventilator, resulting in the patient's death. A *terminal wean* involves slowly decreasing ventilator support so that the patient is receiving less help breathing over time. To avoid the patient experiencing feelings of suffocation and fear, he is simultaneously given medication (often pain medication) for sedation so that he is not aware and not struggling to breathe during this process. It may take hours to wean a patient from the ventilator, and, depending on the patient's respiratory status, he may survive without the ventilator for an additional several hours. During this process patients are not awake and alert, but family members can be with them for their final moments.

EOL decisions are often difficult for the patient and family, but the psychologist is uniquely suited to help individuals weigh the pros and cons of the specific decisions. The clinician can also facilitate discussions with the medical team if patients or families have additional questions. Once the decisions about withdrawing or withholding treatment (or any other aspects of EOL care) are made, any formal orders would be documented in the medical record by the patient's physician. The psychologist should provide documentation on what preceded the decision, such as a summary of family discussions, the results of a capacity assessment, or information on the patient's values that informed the ultimate decision.

SPECIFIC CONCERNS OF RESPIRATORY PATIENTS

Studies of patients with serious lung disease (although not necessarily at the end of their lives) have documented the issues of most concern to them (Bereza, Troelsgaard Nielsen, Valgardsson, Hemels, & Einarson, 2015; Hall, Legault, & Côté, 2010; Rocker, Dodek, & Heyland, 2008); see Exhibit 10.1. These concerns are quite similar to those found in dying patients with nonrespiratory illnesses (e.g., Heyland et al., 2006; Miccinesi, Bianchi, Brunelli, & Borreani, 2012).

The top priority among patients with advanced COPD is that they not be kept on life support if there is no hope of meaningful recovery (Rocker et al., 2008). Symptom relief and control (for breathlessness, cough, sputum production, fatigue, and other symptoms) is also critically important to patients, and they want as little discomfort and symptom impact on their lives as possible. Patients want to be informed about their medical status and treatment options, and they want to maintain control over decisions

EXHIBIT 10.1. Issues of Importance for Pulmonary Patients at End of Life

Not being kept alive needlessly
Symptom relief
Fears of suffocation and panic
Maintaining control over medical decisions
Not being a burden on family
Trust in providers/receiving good care
Being informed
Preparing for death

Note. Data from Bereza, Troelsgaard Nielsen, Valgardsson, Hemels, and Einarson (2015); Hall, Legault, and Côté (2010); Rocker, Dodek, and Heyland (2008).

about their treatment. They want good care to be available to them and trusting relationships with their medical providers. Not burdening loved ones, either with caregiving responsibilities or financial obligations, is also of concern to patients. Many people want to prepare for their deaths by resolving old relationship conflicts, getting their affairs in order, or making funeral and burial plans.

PSYCHOLOGICAL TREATMENT OF PULMONARY PATIENTS AT THE END OF LIFE

The overall goal of psychological intervention is to provide the patient with a "good death" that allows them dignity and comfort, avoids isolation, and is consistent with their wishes (see Beckstrand, Callister, & Kirchhoff, 2006). Exhibit 10.2 is a list of tasks a psychologist might be involved in when treating a patient at the end of her life. These are discussed in more detail below.

Providing Information, Support, and Referral

The psychologist's work with a respiratory patient at EOL may be different from other times in the patient's life; the patient may feel some urgency to address her or his concerns because the remaining time may be short. Further, even if the patient has well-meaning family members, many are unwilling to discuss EOL concerns with the patient. Families often continue to encourage patients to be optimistic and hopeful, even when hope is no longer realistic, and they may be unwilling to discuss a patient's wishes for her funeral or burial. The psychologist can discuss anything on the patient's mind and can encourage him to write down his wishes for family to fulfill later.

EXHIBIT 10.2. Psychological Interventions With End-of-Life (EOL) Respiratory Patients

Support the patient, family, and surrogate decision makers
Monitor psychological symptoms
Intervene with coping skills, relaxation techniques, and other psychological strategies
Provide education about advance directives, psychological impacts of EOL
Refer to other specialists as needed (e.g., chaplain, psychiatry)
Monitor cognition; assess decisional capacity, if warranted
Work as part of the medical team to help the family make decisions
Advocate for the patient with the medical team

Psychologists can provide patients (and family) with information about EOL, grief, advance directives, and other relevant matters, if they so desire. The psychologist can also facilitate discussions with the medical team if the patient has questions about his current medical status so that he can develop realistic expectations. Referrals can also be made to a chaplain if the patient wishes spiritual support or to social work for other matters (e.g., insurance questions).

It has often been thought that people who are dying will want to make amends or complete unfinished business with important others in their lives. For example, this might entail locating a brother who the patient has been estranged from for 20 years, or a child who has not had contact with the patient since moving to a foreign country 5 years ago. For those patients who wish to address matters such as these, the mental health provider can help them consider what such contact might be like (i.e., what the patient's goals are and the likelihood of them being met) and how he would feel if the person did not wish to make contact. Some people, however, will have no wish to revisit old interpersonal issues, and that is acceptable, too. One patient noted, "I haven't spoken to my brother in 10 years, why would I want to talk to him now?"

Monitor and Treat Anxiety, Depression, and Grief

Regardless of the setting, the psychologist will want to monitor the patient's mood and psychological symptoms, using standardized questionnaires, interview, or family observations and reports. Symptoms of anxiety and depression are not unexpected when respiratory patients are facing EOL, and they may be especially problematic if patients have a history of anxiety and depression. Because some psychological symptoms can exacerbate breathlessness and other pulmonary problems, they should be addressed through psychotherapy, medication adjustments, or the prescription of psychotropic medications to alleviate symptoms. (See Chapters 6 and 7, on anxiety and depression, for specific psychological interventions.)

When it is clear that the patient is near the end of her life, both the patient and the family may begin to grieve. Much has been written on the stages of grief (i.e., denial, anger, bargaining, depression, and acceptance; Kübler-Ross, 1969). Individuals usually do not progress neatly through these stages but, instead, go back and forth or may experience more than one aspect at a time. The psychologist can provide support, help people to express and organize their feelings or regrets, and aid in the use of coping strategies to help them manage their emotions during this time.

A special case occurs when the death is of a young person, which occurs often with cystic fibrosis. Patients and families have likely been aware that the patient could die at a young age for a long time, but that does not make it easier when death occurs. Older people and their families may feel the person has lived a good life and may accept death more readily, but this is harder with young people who may not have been able to get married, have children, or develop their careers. This is the patient's loss, but it also impacts the family because they will not see their family member reach milestones such as graduation or marriage. Both patients and family members may benefit from a discussion of the unfairness of the situation and their sadness over events that will not occur.

Dealing With Delirium and Decisional Capacity

Cognition should be monitored because many patients demonstrate cognitive changes as the disease progresses. Delirium is a clinical emergency in which a medical problem causes changes in a patient's behavior or cognition. Common clinical features of delirium are listed in Exhibit 10.3 (more detail is in Labott, 2019). Cognition may be seriously impaired. Families may report that the patient "is not himself" emotionally, and the patient may be unable to remember to take his medication or to care for himself without supervision. Delirious patients may demonstrate poor judgment and be fearful, and, in the hospital, they are at risk of hurting themselves if they decide to escape. Patients may present with behavior that is agitated, hypoactive, or mixed (Liptzin & Levkoff, 1992), and the impairments and symptoms may fluctuate.

Delirium is common in the medically ill elderly, and in respiratory patients, it often occurs secondary to infection, poor oxygen saturation, or coexisting multiple medical problems. Although delirium is theoretically

EXHIBIT 10.3. Clinical Features of Delirium

Changes in attention and awareness
Cognitive changes
Rapid onset
Fluctuating course
Psychotic symptoms
Irrational thinking
Uncharacteristic behavior and emotional reactions
Hyperactivity or hypoactivity
Reversibility

Note. Data from Labott (2019).

reversible as the medical cause is treated, in the context of end-stage disease it may not be possible to reverse the medical problem (e.g., oxygen saturation remains poor in spite of all possible treatment), so the delirium may be ongoing. While the medical team will address the medical causes of the delirium, the psychologist may be involved in plans to keep the patient physically safe and emotionally comfortable. This may involve coordinating the family so that the patient is not alone, educating family and staff on the need to reorient the patient frequently, and reassuring the patient that he is safe. Families may need education so that they understand that the patient's behavior is caused by the medical problem and should be understood in that context. A patient may become angry or verbally abusive with a spouse; a delirious patient should not be viewed as "mean," nor should this be taken as a rift in the relationship. Similarly, a patient's behavior may be atypically oppositional or aggressive; this should not be attributed to personality factors but viewed as a symptom of the delirium.

In the context of cognitive or behavioral changes, a psychologist may be called on to evaluate a patient's decisional capacity. At EOL, this evaluation would determine if a patient is able to make decisions about treatment choices or about withholding or withdrawing life-supporting measures. If the patient does not have decisional capacity, a surrogate will make decisions on the patient's behalf. To maintain decisional capacity, a patient must be able to communicate a choice regarding the decision (even if this is not communicated verbally), demonstrate understanding of the information relevant to the decision, understand the consequences of the decision, and manipulate information to reason about the pros and cons of the decision. Decisional capacity evaluations can be complicated, especially because patients are often unable to communicate easily at this stage of the illness, and repeat evaluations may be necessary as a patient's capacity may change over time. Appelbaum and Grisso (1988), Leo (1999), and Searight (1992) provided classic articles on this process. Detailed procedures for these evaluations and specific interview questions to assess a patient's capacity are found in Labott (2019). Case 10.1 is an example of a patient facing EOL decisions who did not have decisional capacity.

Working With the Medical Team and Advocating for the Patient

Especially in a hospital setting, the psychologist will want to understand the relevant medical issues and work closely with the medical team. Whereas the primary medical providers are responsible for providing medical information to patients, the psychologist may be called on to review information with patients and families and to help them make treatment decisions.

CASE 10.1
DELIRIUM AT END OF LIFE

Mrs. G was a 50-year-old divorced woman, admitted to the hospital with pneumonia, and on a ventilator. The patient had received bilateral lung transplant at age 46 for idiopathic pulmonary fibrosis. She had initially done well but developed chronic rejection (bronchiolitis obliterans) about eight months ago, and she had been on a ventilator for the past 5 months. She was not a candidate for another transplant; rejection had been treated with steroids and other medications, but these were becoming less effective over time. The new pneumonia made the situation bleak.

Mrs. G was mildly sedated, and she had been delirious for the past few days (likely due to the infection); she had been scared and fearful that nurses were trying to hurt her, she had been refusing all medical tests, and she tried to pull out her breathing tube as well as IV lines. The patient's only family was a younger sister who lived 500 miles away but was coming to the hospital today.

The psychologist was consulted because the patient's doctors believed that further treatment was futile. They felt they could make progress on treating the pneumonia, but that this would not buy the patient much quantity or quality time. Prior to development of the pneumonia she had been unable to ambulate or move much at all, spending most of her day on the toilet as it was too difficult for her to walk back and forth when she had to use the bathroom. Beyond the physical limitations, she was in extreme discomfort due to breathlessness, and she slept much of the day and night. Even with ventilator support, it was anticipated that her pulmonary functioning would worsen and that she would continue to deteriorate quickly. The doctors felt that they could keep her alive for a short while, but her time would be of poor quality because if she was alert she would be in significant discomfort due to breathlessness, and if she was sedated she would be unable to interact with others or participate in any activities. They saw no possibility of significant improvement in her medical status.

The request was for the psychologist to evaluate the patient to determine if she understood the situation and was able to make decisions about her treatment. First, plans were made to help the patient be at her best cognitively, that is, she was given her glasses and nurses minimized sedating medication so that she could stay awake. The patient was unable to talk because it took too much energy, but she was able to signal answers to yes-no questions with her finger.

The patient's doctor reviewed her medical situation with her, the expected course, and her impression that further treatment would be

(continues)

CASE 10.1
DELIRIUM AT END OF LIFE (*Continued*)

futile and would only prolong her life a bit, without any improvement in her life quality. This information was provided in lay terms, with the psychologist and the patient's nurse present, and aspects of it were repeated several times, as the patient was somnolent and had to be awakened and refocused repeatedly. When asked, the patient always indicated that she understood the information provided to her, although it was not clear that she did.

After the doctor left, the psychologist began to evaluate the patient to determine her preferences and understanding of the situation. The patient agreed to everything (even when asked the same question in opposite ways, she would always agree, contradicting herself). She was unable to accurately report (through indicating yes or no with her finger) her age, occupation, or medical status. On exam, her mental status was significantly impaired, with problems in orientation, memory, and attention. She alternately agreed and disagreed with the withdrawal of the ventilator and other treatments, and the pattern of her responses indicated that she did not understand. The psychologist attempted to assess other aspects of cognition and mood, although the patient did not seem to understand many of the questions, and she was becoming more and more somnolent, so the interview was kept brief. It was concluded that the patient was not currently capable of making her own decisions, so the plan was to enlist her sister to do so.

When the patient's sister arrived, she spent some time with the patient, and the psychologist again attempted to interview Mrs. G. She behaved similarly to the initial evaluation that morning and did not seem to understand. At one point she reached for the psychologist's pad and pen, wrote the letters J-O-Y, and gave it to her sister. While the writing was difficult for her, the letters could be made out clearly. The patient was unable to explain what she meant by this; her sister felt the patient was happy about going to heaven soon.

The sister then met with the doctor, the psychologist, the patient's nurse, and the hospital chaplain. All the information on the patient's medical status was relayed to her and options were discussed. It was decided that antibiotics and nutrition would be stopped, a DNR order would be written, hydration would continue, and the patient would slowly be weaned from the ventilator, which would likely result in her death over the next few days. The patient's sister wished to remain with the patient during this time.

Over the next 12 hours, the ventilator was slowly withdrawn, and the patient remained sedated and comfortable. Several hours after the ventilator was completely withdrawn, she died peacefully.

The psychologist may also participate in team meetings with doctors, the patient/family/surrogate decision maker, a chaplain, and others to provide information and discuss options for the patient's care.

Psychologists can also be an advocate for the patient at EOL. At times, advocacy might involve a request for the doctor to reevaluate the patient for additional pain medication or for nurses to provide some uninterrupted time for the patient to rest or to talk by phone with a close family member who cannot visit in person. Special arrangements can also be facilitated by the psychologist in an effort to make the patient's quality of life the best it can be. In some instances, the medical team will bend hospital rules, for example, to enable a child who is under the allowed visiting age to visit the patient or to get the patient his favorite food, even if it is something he is not allowed to have.

Supporting Family and Surrogates

At some point, the patient may no longer be alert or responsive, so the psychologist will not be able to intervene with her directly. However, the psychologist should continue to monitor the patient for changes, with special attention to the patient's comfort. If the patient does not appear quiet and comfortable, that should be addressed with the medical team. At this phase of the patient's life, education and support of family members or surrogates may become the priority, with additional psychological intervention (e.g., coping strategies) or referrals provided to them as needed.

After the death, family members will grieve the loss. If a clinician continues treatment with a family member, she can be educated about the fact that grief can last a long time, even though many believe they should be "over it" in a year. They can also be educated about other psychological problems, especially depression, and when to seek additional treatment if they are not progressing through the grief process. People need to understand there is no "fix" for grief, but support and time will help them to gain a new perspective and move on (without forgetting their family member). Individual treatment or support groups can be useful for family members during this time.

EMOTIONAL IMPACTS ON THE PSYCHOLOGIST

Many psychologists are uncomfortable with EOL treatment issues initially but become more comfortable with experience. As with many other problems facing seriously ill patients, there is no way the psychologist can remedy the situation. Because this work can be stressful and emotionally draining, providers will need to be attentive to their own self-care.

The psychologist's reaction to the loss of a patient will not be the same for all but will be largely determined by the specific relationship the provider had with a particular patient. Addressing grief will involve an awareness of one's own emotional reactions and attention to ways it can influence inter-actions with patients or personal relationships. Consulting with colleagues is often a useful way to obtain help to manage the grief. Especially if the psychologist has a caseload in which repeated losses occur over a short period of time, a group of professionals who meet regularly to discuss these issues can be helpful. Dwyer, Deshields, and Nanna (2012) suggested the use of a "grief ritual," a behavior the psychologist uses to acknowledge or commemorate the loss, such as a prayer or a time for reflection. As with other professional issues, psychologists will want to continue to monitor and address their own emotional state to ensure they are at their best to treat other patients.

11 ETHICS AND PROFESSIONAL ISSUES

Psychologists have much to offer to respiratory patients. The importance of evaluation, treatment, and collaboration with medical teams has been discussed throughout this book. Psychologists are also well positioned to work on the prevention of pulmonary disease, both with individual patients and in the context of larger public health programs. Finally, psychologists in research settings continue to provide empirical data on psychological factors that affect respiratory disease as well as effective interventions for this group.

The *Ethical Principles of Psychologists and Code of Conduct* (American Psychological Association [APA], 2017a; hereinafter, APA Ethics Code) pertains to all of this work. The *Guidelines for Psychological Practice in Health Care Delivery Systems* (APA, 2013) also address ethical behavior for psychologists working with medical patients and speak to issues such as professional identity, the psychologist's role, and collaborative care. Another helpful resource is a chapter by Hanson, Kerkhoff, and Bush (2005) on the ethical care of medical outpatients that includes useful case examples. There are some specific challenges that can occur when treating medical patients, for example, confidentiality is more complicated when working

http://dx.doi.org/10.1037/0000189-012
Psychological Treatment of Patients With Chronic Respiratory Disease, by S. M. Labott

with family members and medical teams than when working with the patient alone. This and other professional and ethical challenges are described below.

DEVELOPING A PRACTICE WITH RESPIRATORY PATIENTS

Pulmonologists and other physicians are often eager for the help of a psychologist because they are aware of how psychological symptoms can interfere with the patient's medical treatment. Yet, they may be unaware of mental health providers who have the expertise to treat respiratory patients. In some settings, it may only require the psychologist to call a few colleagues to let them know she is available to see these patients, but in other settings it is more difficult, and psychologists may need to actively market their services.

The psychologist will need to carefully consider the services that he can provide, for example, outpatient evaluation, ongoing behavioral medicine treatment, inpatient consultation, family work, or all of the above. The content of the marketing materials should then focus on the specific services to be provided. Brochures are one way to target the patient, the doctor, or both. They should explain the psychological services provided, including information on how these services are useful for the patient and the physician. They should include some background information on the psychologist and information on the office location and how to schedule an appointment. In some cases, additional information can be helpful (e.g., languages other than English spoken, insurances accepted). Brochures can be educational for the medical staff and can then be given to the patient by the doctor when the situation warrants it. Adding a personal touch can help with referrals—perhaps a psychologist can call ahead and request a few minutes of the doctor's time to introduce herself when delivering the brochures (and it will help the developing relationship if this is kept to only a few minutes).

Another way to become known to physicians is to provide them with education on the issues that a psychologist can address to improve the patient's quality of life (e.g., treating depression) and/or to help the medical staff manage aspects of the patient's care more successfully (e.g., how to improve adherence). In large medical centers, a psychologist could perhaps deliver a Grand Rounds presentation to physicians. In smaller practice settings, the psychologist could do a short presentation to the doctor's office staff about a specific topic they may struggle with in their work (e.g., dealing with anxious patients). In either case, the medical team will gain a broader perspective on how to use the expertise of the psychologist.

It may also be necessary to explicitly educate medical providers and their staff about the role that a psychologist can play in the care of pulmonary patients. Those who have not worked with psychologists before may expect a psychologist to deal exclusively with traditional psychopathology and may need education about the broader role that a psychologist can play, for example, in adherence or in end-of-life (EOL) issues. Some medical providers may not be aware of the distinction between a psychologist and a psychiatrist or between a psychologist and a social worker.

Many patients referred to psychologists never make it to the psychologist's office, so anything that can be done to make it easier for patients is desirable. Suggesting an approach to the referral of patients can be helpful, regardless of the setting. It is often most useful for the medical provider to present the psychologist as a member of the treatment team who will help the patient to cope with the medical problem and to maximize the impact of the medical treatment. A low-key approach that does *not* label the individual as a psychiatric patient is most useful and elicits little resistance from most patients.

For those affiliated with a medical center, at times the psychologist can see the patient in the medical clinic (at least initially), because that location is typically more comfortable and more within the patient's frame of reference than attending a mental health clinic. If the psychologist is well integrated into the pulmonary clinic, she may have established hours to see patients there, for example, one day weekly. (These arrangements, however, depend on available space and other factors.) Even in a small medical practice, it may be possible to schedule the psychologist to meet briefly with the patient at his next visit to the doctor's office. If patients need to be seen at the psychologist's office, they are more likely to comply if the medical staff can schedule an appointment for them, providing directions and other instructions.

After receiving a referral, the psychologist will want to be sure he understands the referral question, so he may need a brief conversation with the referral source to clarify any questions. The referral source can often provide valuable behavioral data to help the psychologist in formulating a plan for the evaluation. Common referral concerns for respiratory patients include anxiety, depression, nonadherence, cognitive changes, problems coping, and EOL concerns (see also Exhibit 4.1 in Chapter 4).

Prior to the initial visit, the psychologist will want to review background information on the patient. If the psychologist and the referral source are part of the same hospital or practice, the psychologist can generally access the patient's medical records to obtain a detailed history. If not, the referral source can provide some background verbally or by providing written reports or a summary of the patient's care. Usually the more information, the better, but if the psychologist has at least some idea of the patient's medical and psychological history, much of the detail can be obtained from the patient or the family at the time of the initial evaluation.

Providing feedback to the referral source is not only a critical part of patient care, but much informal education occurs when the psychologist explains the conclusions and recommendations and provides additional information about the role she can play in the patient's ongoing treatment. The written report should be thorough but concise and summarize the evaluation including relevant conclusions and recommendations.

In many cases, the referring physician may also want a brief verbal report soon after the patient's initial evaluation. A verbal report will include the main conclusions about the patient's current psychological symptoms and relevant psychiatric history, cognitive status, an opinion on the referral question, and any recommendations. The psychologist will need to be clear about which recommendations she will address (e.g., brief therapy to improve adherence) versus those that she is asking the physician to perform (e.g., review the patient's medications and their purposes with him, order neuropsychological testing). Through this process, the psychologist can also demonstrate her role and the usefulness of the information obtained to improve the patient's ongoing care and psychological adjustment.

The psychologist needs to determine up front what feedback is preferred by the specific referring physician. Further, the psychologist should know how and when the physician wants feedback when treatment is ongoing; for example, some physicians prefer an update on the psychological treatment every few months, whereas others only request a call from the psychologist if there is new information about which she should be aware.

THE PSYCHOLOGIST'S ROLE AND PROFESSIONAL IDENTITY

The psychologist who works with respiratory patients will want to develop a unique identity as an independent member of the treatment team (APA, 2013, Guideline 3) with special expertise in psychopathology, behavior change, and biopsychosocial conceptualization and treatment. The psychologist can perform several roles in the treatment of the respiratory patient. As a *consultant*, the psychologist may evaluate the patient, providing recommendations for the treatment team, with little or no further personal contact with the patient. The psychologist may play the role of an *educator* for the patient, family, and medical treatment providers, providing information about expected reactions to a diagnosis of pulmonary disease, psychological symptoms and their interaction with respiratory symptoms, and interventions to aid the patient's coping and adjustment. The psychologist may also serve as a *therapist* for the patient, providing traditional weekly intervention sessions (including the family as warranted) and intervening from a biopsychosocial perspective. Alternatively, the therapy may occur in nontraditional ways, for example, a psychologist could see the patient when he arrives for his visit with the pulmonologist every few months to provide ongoing monitoring and brief interventions. The goals of all these roles are to promote adjustment, adaptive behavior change, and improvement in the patient's quality of life.

Respect and credibility with medical providers are largely obtained as the psychologist demonstrates a firm knowledge of respiratory physiology, diseases, and treatments; overlap with psychological symptoms; and psychological interventions to improve the patient's adjustment, adherence, and overall life quality. Medical providers expect the psychologist to understand the relevant medical issues so that they can develop an accurate biopsychosocial conceptualization and then provide intervention through psychological methods. A caveat, however: No matter the psychologist's background in understanding respiratory disease, all patients are different, and the psychologist should not hesitate to ask questions of medical personnel regarding information that is unclear.

The psychologist needs to have an understanding of the roles and expertise of the other medical professionals involved in the patient's care to work collaboratively with them. Knowledge about the background and specific activities of pulmonary rehabilitation nurses, pulmonary function technicians, and others will help the psychologist to understand the patient's experiences and enable more effective interaction with these other professionals.

CONFIDENTIALITY

It is a general ethical principle that information shared by clients with the psychologist is confidential; in the evaluation and treatment of medical patients, however, there are often limits to confidentiality of which a patient needs to be aware. When treating a respiratory patient, information may be shared with the patient's doctor and other members of the treatment team. If family members are involved in the patient's care, certain information may also be shared with them. Patients will need to know and agree to the limits of confidentiality when meeting with the psychologist, consistent with the APA Ethics Code (2017a, Ethical Standard 4.02, Discussing the Limits of Confidentiality). Typically, patients need to understand that a summary of their evaluation or treatment will be provided to their doctor verbally, in writing, or both. (A signed release from the patient may be required for this purpose.)

The involvement of family members can be important with respiratory patients, and the psychologist and patient need to agree on what information will be shared with them. The psychologist will want the patient's permission to involve family members in the evaluation or treatment. Some patients are happy to have a spouse or significant other involved in all aspects of their psychological care, and others are comfortable, for example, with a daughter providing some history but do not want her to be aware of emotional issues discussed with the psychologist. These arrangements need to be clear to all parties. Case 11.1 demonstrates how the limits to confidentiality can be managed in the case of a patient who wanted specific information withheld from her doctor and family.

COMPETENCE

Core competencies have been proposed for clinical psychologists and include skills such as assessment, intervention, consultation, and knowledge about ethics and cultural issues (e.g., DiTomasso, Cahn, Panichelli-Mindel, & McFillin, 2013). Additional competencies have been described for psychologists working in medical settings. These include (a) Assessment: knowledge of measures appropriate for medical conditions and an understanding of the possible effects of medical symptoms and medications on standard psychological measures, (b) Advocacy: regarding a patient's needs and also available services, (c) Teaching: educating medical personnel about the biopsychosocial model, and (d) Professionalism: the need for continuing education as well as an ability to deal appropriately with medical patients (Dobmeyer & Rowan, 2014). The extent to which a psychologist needs to develop competency in each of these areas will depend on the setting, the patient population, and the types of services offered by the psychologist.

With respect to the practicalities of working with respiratory patients, specifically, there are a variety of resources available to inform the work of the psychologist. Certain websites (e.g., https://webmd.com and https://mayoclinic.org) are good resources on specific respiratory symptoms and

CASE 11.1
MANAGING CONFIDENTIALITY CONCERNS

Mrs. T was a 55-year-old married woman, referred by her internist for the evaluation and management of anxiety that seemed secondary to a new diagnosis of chronic obstructive pulmonary disease. The psychologist was also asked to meet with the patient's husband and grown children to provide education on adjustment and support.

The patient attended the evaluation alone and was informed of the limits of confidentiality, including that a summary report would be provided to her doctor and that some information would be shared with her family in the later meeting. She had no problems with that.

A typical biopsychosocial evaluation was performed and included a discussion of the patient's social situation, medical issues, substance use, psychological history and current status, and a brief mental status examination. Mrs. T did report new problems with anxiety since her diagnosis, and the specifics of the anxiety were thoroughly delineated.

In the course of the evaluation, the patient noted several pieces of information that she did not want shared with her doctor or her family. These included (a) she had a brief affair about ten years ago, (b) she had used cocaine on occasion in her 30s, and (c) she was regularly taking Valium from her sister's prescription. She was unaware of the dose. The psychologist agreed that the affair and the cocaine use could be left out of the information shared with the doctor and her family. He also agreed that the family did not need to know about the Valium use but felt that the patient's doctor did need to know this information. The patient became angry, noting that the psychologist had told her that her doctor would receive a report, but she didn't feel that this was relevant to her medical treatment and so could be left out.

The psychologist described how a drug such as Valium was quite relevant to her medical treatment because it could possibly decrease her respiratory drive, therefore increasing breathing problems, and it could also possibly interact with her other medications, creating side effects or decreasing their usefulness. The psychologist explained that while the extent of the potential problems would likely depend on the dose of the medication she was taking, these issues were important not only for the treatment of her pulmonary disease but could also be a safety concern.

The patient began to cry, noting that she was just trying to "deal with things" and didn't want her doctor to think she was a bad person. The psychologist empathized with her difficulty coping with these new changes in her life. He noted this is not about her being a bad person, but that her doctor would want her to feel better physically and emotionally, and that

(continues)

CASE 11.1

MANAGING CONFIDENTIALITY CONCERNS (*Continued*)

he could help her find more adaptive ways to feel better. He suggested that perhaps it would be OK with her doctor if she continued the medication, but then he could consider this in the overall treatment of her disease, or perhaps it would be better for him to provide a different medication to help with her anxiety that would be safer. The psychologist indicated that he would also work with the patient on anxiety management and described the use of relaxation, cognitive strategies, and distraction. The patient was comfortable with this treatment plan and also participated in a brief relaxation procedure, which she felt good about.

Afterward, the patient agreed that the information about her Valium use could be shared with her doctor, but not with her family. She was also instructed to not abruptly stop the Valium, but to return to her doctor to discuss what should be done about this. She agreed to return weekly for a few weeks to see the psychologist about anxiety management, and the family meeting was scheduled. Afterward, the psychologist called her doctor with a verbal report of the main findings of the evaluation and the treatment plan (consistent with the agreements about confidentiality developed with the patient) and followed this with a written report.

The next week the family meeting went well. The patient was also able to meet with her doctor the following week. He felt the dose of Valium that she was taking was too high, so they developed a plan to slowly wean her off of it, and he planned to then replace it with a safer medication. Mrs. T continued to work with the psychologist for a few more weeks on anxiety management strategies. By the end of the psychological treatment, she had begun taking Buspar (which she was tolerating well), and she was consistently using relaxation and cognitive anxiety management strategies. Her anxiety was minimal generally, and she was able to manage episodes of increased anxiety successfully.

disorders. The Global Initiative for Chronic Obstructive Lung Disease (GOLD, 2018) and The Global Initiative for Asthma (GINA, 2018) provide extensive information on current diagnostic testing, medical treatments, comorbidities, and other important facts about chronic obstructive pulmonary disease and asthma, respectively. Psychologists can also review professional journals and attend medical conferences dedicated to respiratory disease to keep abreast of new developments in medical treatments. The American Thoracic Society (ATS) has an annual conference that includes presentations on psychological issues in respiratory disease. ATS also has a website (http://thoracic.org)

that provides a wealth of information, including guidelines for the medical treatment of many respiratory diseases.

Competence may also be demonstrated formally by obtaining certification in clinical health psychology by the American Board of Professional Psychology (https://abpp.org). The process of board certification takes time and effort, but it does formally document a psychologist's competence in working with medical patients. In addition, board certification is viewed positively by physicians, as it is similar to their own boarding process.

CULTURE AND DIVERSITY

The APA Ethics Code (2017a, Ethical Standard 2.01b, Boundaries of Competence) requires an understanding of issues of culture and diversity, such as race, gender, socioeconomic status, religion, ethnicity, sexual orientation, and other factors, and particularly the impact of these factors on a patient's psychological evaluation and treatment. The Multicultural Guidelines (APA, 2017b) provide specific guidance on the importance of understanding the role of culture in the individual's identity and interactions with others, as well as the psychologist's need to understand his or her assumptions and provide culturally appropriate treatment.

There are differences in the prevalence of pulmonary diseases that are based on gender and race (see Chapter 3). Most chronic respiratory diseases occur more frequently in older people, with some exceptions (e.g., cystic fibrosis). Although the symptoms of pulmonary disease, the experience of breathlessness, and associated physical limitations are similar across diverse groups, an individual's reactions to them may differ, largely on the basis of the interpretation of the meaning of the symptom or disease. Cultural beliefs about a disease, its cause, and treatments can influence the patient's adherence, support-seeking, and expectations of providers; medical belief systems and cultural values can also play a significant role in the disease course and medical outcomes (e.g., Karel, 2007; Sussman, 2004, 2008).

There are steps a psychologist can take to ensure that he is appropriately mindful of culture and diversity factors. Having a general understanding of some of the varieties of cultural beliefs about health care can provide a context from which to understand new patients. Clear communication with a patient is then critically important. This will involve making the patient comfortable enough to discuss any cultural factors that may be relevant. Good communication may also require the use of an interpreter or other aids so that the psychologist clearly understands what the patient is trying to communicate. Finally, the psychologist should not hesitate simply to *ask* the patient about his understanding and interpretations of specific information relevant to the psychological or medical treatment.

PSYCHOLOGICAL TREATMENT OF RESPIRATORY PATIENTS

Patients with chronic respiratory diseases may struggle with physiological challenges (e.g., shortness of breath) as well as psychological challenges (e.g., anxiety or depression). Psychologists who understand respiratory disease can apply traditional evidence-based psychological intervention strategies to provide significant benefits for pulmonary patients. One of the challenges in working with pulmonary patients involves the need to continually be mindful of the medical problem, so that adjustments may be made in the psychological treatment (e.g., avoiding interventions that will tax the patient's respiratory system). Such adjustments can ensure the psychological treatment is both safe and effective for the patient.

With these caveats in mind, psychologists can provide a variety of services to pulmonary patients, including evaluation, outpatient psychotherapy, inpatient consultation, or family intervention. The interventions can help patients to be more active and productive, maintain important social relationships, manage their medical regimen, cope with their disease and treatment, and improve their overall quality of life. Although there are challenges for the psychologist, it is quite rewarding to see how resilient and motivated respiratory patients can be in spite of significant impacts on their psychological and physical functioning.

References

Adegunsoye, A., Strek, M. E., Garrity, E., Guzy, R., & Bag, R. (2017). Comprehensive care of the lung transplant patient. *Chest, 152*, 150–164. http://dx.doi.org/10.1016/j.chest.2016.10.001

Ágh, T., Inotai, A., & Mészáros, Á. (2011). Factors associated with medication adherence in patients with chronic obstructive pulmonary disease. *International Review of Thoracic Diseases, 82*, 328–334. http://dx.doi.org/10.1159/000324453

Agrawal, S., & Britton, J. R. (2017). Smoking cessation. In G. P. Currie (Ed.), *ABC of COPD* (3rd ed., pp. 27–33). Newark, NJ: John Wiley & Sons.

Ahuja, J., Kanne, J. P., & Meyer, C. A. (2015). Occupational lung disease. *Seminars in Roentgenology, 50*, 40–51. http://dx.doi.org/10.1053/j.ro.2014.04.010

Alexis-Garsee, C., Gilbert, H., Burton, M., & van den Akker, O. (2018). Difficulties quitting for smokers with and without a respiratory disease and use of a tailored intervention for smoking cessation—A qualitative study. *Journal of Smoking Cessation, 13*, 63–71. http://dx.doi.org/10.1017/jsc.2017.5

Alexopoulos, G. S., Sirey, J. A., Banerjee, S., Kiosses, D. N., Pollari, C., Novitch, R. S., . . . Raue, P. J. (2016). Two behavioral interventions for patients with major depression and severe COPD. *The American Journal of Geriatric Psychiatry, 24*, 964–974. http://dx.doi.org/10.1016/j.jagp.2016.07.014

American Lung Association. (n.d.). *Clean air*. Retrieved from http://www.cleanairchoice.org/air/

American Psychological Association. (2013). Guidelines for psychological practice in health care delivery systems. *American Psychologist, 68*(1), 1–6. Retrieved from https://www.apa.org/pubs/journals/features/delivery-systems.pdf

American Psychological Association. (2017a). *Ethical principles of psychologists and code of conduct* (2002, amended June 1, 2010, and January 1, 2017). Retrieved from http://www.apa.org/ethics/code/ethics-code-2017.pdf

American Psychological Association. (2017b). *Multicultural guidelines: An ecological approach to context, identity, and intersectionality*. Retrieved from http://www.apa.org/about/policy/multicultural-guidelines.pdf

American Sleep Association (ASA). (2019). *Sleep and sleep disorder statistics.* Retrieved from https://www.sleepassociation.org/about-sleep/sleep-statistics/

Andenaes, R., Kalfoss, M. H., & Wahl, A. K. (2006). Coping and psychological distress in hospitalized patients with chronic obstructive pulmonary disease. *Heart & Lung, 35,* 46–57. http://dx.doi.org/10.1016/j.hrtlng.2005.09.009

Andrianopoulos, V., Gloeckl, R., Vogiatzis, I., & Kenn, K. (2017). Cognitive impairment in COPD: Should cognitive evaluation be part of respiratory assessment? *Breathe, 13,* e1–e9. http://dx.doi.org/10.1183/20734735.001417

Anstiss, T., & Passmore, J. (2012). Motivational interviewing. *Cognitive behavioural coaching in practice: An evidence based approach* (pp. 33–52). New York, NY: Routledge/Taylor & Francis Group, New York, NY.

Appelbaum, P. S., & Grisso, T. (1988). Assessing patients' capacities to consent to treatment. *The New England Journal of Medicine, 319,* 1635–1638. http://dx.doi.org/10.1056/NEJM198812223192504

Apter, A. J., Boston, R. C., George, M., Norfleet, A. L., Tenhave, T., Coyne, J. C., . . . Feldman, H. I. (2003). Modifiable barriers to adherence to inhaled steroids among adults with asthma: It's not just black and white. *The Journal of Allergy and Clinical Immunology, 111,* 1219–1226. http://dx.doi.org/10.1067/mai.2003.1479

Arozullah, A. M., Yarnold, P. R., Bennett, C. L., Soltysik, R. C., Wolf, M. S., Ferreira, R. M., . . . Davis, T. (2007). Development and validation of a short-form, rapid estimate of adult literacy in medicine. *Medical Care, 45,* 1026–1033. http://dx.doi.org/10.1097/MLR.0b013e3180616c1b

Atlantis, E., Fahey, P., Cochrane, B., & Smith, S. (2013). Bidirectional associations between clinically relevant depression or anxiety and COPD: A systematic review and meta-analysis. *Chest, 144,* 766–777. http://dx.doi.org/10.1378/chest.12-1911

Bai, J. W., Chen, X. X., Liu, S., Yu, L., & Xu, J. F. (2017). Smoking cessation affects the natural history of COPD. *International Journal of Chronic Obstructive Pulmonary Disease, 12,* 3323–3328. http://dx.doi.org/10.2147/COPD.S150243

Bandura, A. (1997). *Self-efficacy: The exercise of control.* New York, NY: W. H. Freeman.

Barton, C., Effing, T. W., & Cafarella, P. (2015). Social support and social networks in COPD: A scoping review. *COPD, 12,* 690–702.

Battaglia, S., Bezzi, M., & Sferrazza Papa, G. F. (2014). Are benzodiazepines and opioids really safe in patients with severe COPD? *Minerva Medica, 105* (6 Suppl. 3), 1–7.

Baur, X., & Bakehe, P. (2014). Allergens causing occupational asthma: An evidence-based evaluation of the literature. *International Archives of Occupational and Environmental Health, 87,* 339–363. http://dx.doi.org/10.1007/s00420-013-0866-9

Beck, A. T., Rush, A. J., Shaw, B. F., & Emery, G. (1979). *Cognitive therapy of depression.* New York, NY: Guilford Press.

Beck, A. T., Steer, R. A., & Brown, G. (1996). *Beck depression inventory–II.* http://dx.doi.org/10.1037/t00742-000

Beckstrand, R. L., Callister, L. C., & Kirchhoff, K. T. (2006). Providing a "good death": Critical care nurses' suggestions for improving end-of-life care. *American Journal of Critical Care, 15,* 38–45.

Beernaert, K., Cohen, J., Deliens, L., Devroey, D., Vanthomme, K., Pardon, K., & Van den Block, L. (2013). Referral to palliative care in COPD and other chronic diseases: A population-based study. *Respiratory Medicine, 107,* 1731–1739. http://dx.doi.org/10.1016/j.rmed.2013.06.003

Bereza, B. G., Troelsgaard Nielsen, A., Valgardsson, S., Hemels, M. E., & Einarson, T. R. (2015). Patient preferences in severe COPD and asthma: A comprehensive literature review. *International Journal of Chronic Obstructive Pulmonary Disease, 10,* 739–744. http://dx.doi.org/10.2147/COPD.S82179

Blackley, D. J., Halldin, C. N., & Laney, A. S. (2018). Continued increase in prevalence of coal workers' pneumoconiosis in the United States, 1970–2017. *American Journal of Public Health, 108,* 1220–1222. http://dx.doi.org/10.2105/AJPH.2018.304517

Boé, D. M., Vandivier, R. W., Burnham, E. L., & Moss, M. (2009). Alcohol abuse and pulmonary disease. *Journal of Leukocyte Biology, 86,* 1097–1104. http://dx.doi.org/10.1189/jlb.0209087

Boettcher, H., Brake, C. A., & Barlow, D. H. (2016). Origins and outlook of interoceptive exposure. *Journal of Behavior Therapy and Experimental Psychiatry, 53,* 41–51. http://dx.doi.org/10.1016/j.jbtep.2015.10.009

Bomba, P. A., Kemp, M., & Black, J. S. (2012). POLST: An improvement over traditional advance directives. *Cleveland Clinic Journal of Medicine, 79,* 457–464. http://dx.doi.org/10.3949/ccjm.79a.11098

Borson, S., & Curtis, J. R. (2001). Examining the link between sarcoidosis and depression. *American Journal of Respiratory and Critical Care Medicine, 163,* 306–308. http://dx.doi.org/10.1164/ajrccm.163.2.ed2000b

Borup, H., Kirkeskov, L., Hanskov, D. J. A., & Brauer, C. (2017). Systematic review: Chronic obstructive pulmonary disease and construction workers. *Occupational Medicine, 67,* 199–204. http://dx.doi.org/10.1093/occmed/kqx007

Boudreau, M., Lavoie, K. L., Cartier, A., Trutshnigg, B., Morizio, A., Lemière, C., & Bacon, S. L. (2015). Do asthma patients with panic disorder really have worse asthma? A comparison of physiological and psychological responses to a methacholine challenge. *Respiratory Medicine, 109,* 1250–1256. http://dx.doi.org/10.1016/j.rmed.2015.09.002

Bourbeau, J., & Bartlett, S. J. (2008). Patient adherence in COPD. *Thorax, 63,* 831–838. http://dx.doi.org/10.1136/thx.2007.086041

Bourne, E. J. (2015). *The anxiety and phobia workbook* (6th ed.). Oakland, CA: New Harbinger.

Boustani, M., Peterson, B., Harris, R., Lux, L. J., Krasnov, C., Sutton, S. F., . . . Lohr, K. N. (2003, June). *Screening for dementia.* Rockville, MD: Agency for

Healthcare Research and Quality. Retrieved from https://www.ncbi.nlm.nih.gov/books/NBK42773/

Bragadottir, G. H., Halldorsdottir, B. S., Ingadottir, T. S., & Jonsdottir, H. (2018). Patients and families realising their future with chronic obstructive pulmonary disease—A qualitative study. *Journal of Clinical Nursing, 27,* 57–64. http://dx.doi.org/10.1111/jocn.13843

Braido, F., Chrystyn, H., Baiardini, I., Bosnic-Anticevich, S., van der Molen, T., Dandurand, R. J., . . . Price, D. (2016). "Trying, but failing"—The role of inhaler technique and mode of delivery in respiratory medication adherence. *The Journal of Allergy and Clinical Immunology: In Practice, 4,* 823–832. http://dx.doi.org/10.1016/j.jaip.2016.03.002

Brandstetter, S., Finger, T., Fischer, W., Brandl, M., Böhmer, M., Pfeifer, M., & Apfelbacher, C. (2017). Differences in medication adherence are associated with beliefs about medicines in asthma and COPD. *Clinical and Translational Allergy, 7.* http://dx.doi.org/10.1186/s13601-017-0175-6

Bravo, G., & Hébert, R. (1997). Age- and education-specific reference values for the Mini-Mental and modified Mini-Mental State Examinations derived from a non-demented elderly population. *International Journal of Geriatric Psychiatry, 12,* 1008–1018. http://dx.doi.org/10.1002/(SICI)1099-1166(199710)12:10%3C1008::AID-GPS676%3E3.0.CO;2-A

Brito, L. (2002). *A Saúde mental dos prestadores de cuidados a familiares idosos* [*The Saude mental providers of care to elderly relatives*]. Coimbra, Portugal: Quarteto Editora.

Burns, G. (2017). Chronic obstructive pulmonary disease. In V. Gibson & D. Waters (Eds.), *Respiratory care* (pp. 59–71). Boca Raton, FL: CRC Press/Taylor & Francis.

Cadeddu, C., Capizzi, S., Colombo, D., Nica, M., & De Belvis, A. G. (2016). Literature review of gender differences in respiratory conditions: A focus on asthma and chronic obstructive pulmonary disease (COPD). *Igiene e Sanita Pubblica, 72,* 481–504.

Canino, G., McQuaid, E. L., & Rand, C. S. (2009). Addressing asthma health disparities: A multilevel challenge. *The Journal of Allergy and Clinical Immunology, 123,* 1209–1217. http://dx.doi.org/10.1016/j.jaci.2009.02.043

Cazzola, M., Calzetta, L., Matera, M. G., Hanania, N. A., & Rogliani, P. (2018). How does race/ethnicity influence pharmacological response to asthma therapies? *Expert Opinion on Drug Metabolism & Toxicology, 14,* 435–446. http://dx.doi.org/10.1080/17425255.2018.1449833

Cecere, L. M., Slatore, C. G., Uman, J. E., Evans, L. E., Udris, E. M., Bryson, C. L., & Au, D. H. (2012). Adherence to long-acting inhaled therapies among patients with chronic obstructive pulmonary disease (COPD). *COPD, 9,* 251–258. http://dx.doi.org/10.3109/15412555.2011.650241

Centers for Disease Control and Prevention. (2019a, May). Asthma: Most recent asthma data. Retrieved from https://www.cdc.gov/asthma/most_recent_data.htm

Centers for Disease Control and Prevention. (2019b). Smoking & tobacco use: Current cigarette smoking among adults in the United States. Retrieved from https://www.cdc.gov/tobacco/data_statistics/fact_sheets/adult_data/cig_smoking/index.htm

Centers for Disease Control and Prevention. (2019c). Smoking & tobacco use: Outbreak of lung injury associated with the use of e-cigarette, or vaping, products. Retrieved from https://www.cdc.gov/tobacco/basic_information/e-cigarettes/severe-lung-disease.html

Charles, M. S., Blanchette, C. M., Silver, H., Lavallee, D., Dalal, A. A., & Mapel, D. (2010). Adherence to controller therapy for chronic obstructive pulmonary disease: A review. *Current Medical Research and Opinion, 26,* 2421–2429. http://dx.doi.org/10.1185/03007995.2010.516284

Chaudhary, B. A., Taft, A., & Mishoe, S. C. (2016). Sleep-disordered breathing. In D. R. Hess, N. R. MacIntyre, W. F. Galvin, & S. C. Mishoe (Eds.), *Respiratory care: Principles and practice* (3rd ed., pp. 1033–1052). Burlington, MA: Jones & Bartlett Learning.

Chen, Z., Fan, V. S., Belza, B., Pike, K., & Nguyen, H. Q. (2017). Association between social support and self-care behaviors in adults with chronic obstructive pulmonary disease. *Annals of the American Thoracic Society, 14,* 1419–1427. http://dx.doi.org/10.1513/AnnalsATS.201701-026OC

Chin, K., & Channick, R. N. (2016). Pulmonary hypertension. In V. C. Broaddus, R. J. Mason, J. D. Ernst, T. E. King Jr., S. C. Lazarus, J. F. Murray, . . . M. B. Gotway (Eds.), *Murray & Nadel's textbook of respiratory medicine* (6th ed., pp. 1031–1049.e4). Philadelphia, PA: Elsevier. http://dx.doi.org/10.1016/B978-1-4557-3383-5.00058-0

Choi, J. Y., Chung, H. I., & Han, G. (2014). Patient outcomes according to COPD action plan adherence. *Journal of Clinical Nursing, 23,* 883–891. http://dx.doi.org/10.1111/jocn.12293

Chrystyn, H., Small, M., Milligan, G., Higgins, V., Gil, E. G., & Estruch, J. (2014). Impact of patients' satisfaction with their inhalers on treatment compliance and health status in COPD. *Respiratory Medicine, 108,* 358–365. http://dx.doi.org/10.1016/j.rmed.2013.09.021

Ciprandi, G., Schiavetti, I., Rindone, E., & Ricciardolo, F. L. (2015). The impact of anxiety and depression on outpatients with asthma. *Annals of Allergy, Asthma & Immunology, 115,* 408–414. http://dx.doi.org/10.1016/j.anai.2015.08.007

Cleven, K. L., Webber, M. P., Zeig-Owens, R., Hena, K. M., & Prezant, D. J. (2017). Airway disease in rescue/recovery workers: Recent findings from the World Trade Center collapse. *Current Allergy and Asthma Reports, 17,* 5. http://dx.doi.org/10.1007/s11882-017-0670-9

Clinical Practice Guideline Treating Tobacco Use and Dependence 2008 Update Panel, Liaisons, and Staff (CPG). (2008). A clinical practice guideline for treating tobacco use and dependence: 2008 update. A U.S. public health service report. *American Journal of Preventive Medicine, 35,* 158–176. http://dx.doi.org/10.1016/j.amepre.2008.04.009

Colón, E. A., & Popkin, M. K. (2002). Anxiety and panic. In M. G. Wise & J. R. Rundell (Eds.), *The American Psychiatric Publishing textbook of consultation-liaison psychiatry: Psychiatry in the medically ill* (2nd ed., pp. 393–415). Washington, DC: American Psychiatric Publishing.

Connolly, M. J., & Yohannes, A. M. (2016). The impact of depression in older patients with chronic obstructive pulmonary disease and asthma. *Maturitas, 92*, 9–14. http://dx.doi.org/10.1016/j.maturitas.2016.07.005

Corder, K. (2017). Asthma. In V. Gibson & D. Waters (Eds.), *Respiratory care* (pp. 73–83). Boca Raton, FL: CRC Press/Taylor & Francis.

Cowie, M. R. (2017). Sleep apnea: State of the art. *Trends in Cardiovascular Medicine, 27*, 280–289. http://dx.doi.org/10.1016/j.tcm.2016.12.005

Cruz, I., Marciel, K. K., Quittner, A. L., & Schechter, M. S. (2009). Anxiety and depression in cystic fibrosis. *Seminars in Respiratory and Critical Care Medicine, 30*, 569–578. http://dx.doi.org/10.1055/s-0029-1238915

Cuijpers, P., Vogelzangs, N., Twisk, J., Kleiboer, A., Li, J., & Penninx, B. W. (2014). Comprehensive meta-analysis of excess mortality in depression in the general community versus patients with specific illnesses. *The American Journal of Psychiatry, 171*, 453–462. http://dx.doi.org/10.1176/appi.ajp.2013.13030325

Cullinan, P., Munoz, X., Suojalehto, H., Agius, R., Jindal, S., Sigsgaard, T., . . . Moitra, S. (2017). Occupational lung diseases: From old and novel exposures to effective preventive strategies. *The Lancet: Respiratory Medicine, 5*, 445–455. http://dx.doi.org/10.1016/S2213-2600(16)30424-6

Curtis, L. (2017). Respiratory history taking and physical assessment. *Respiratory care* (pp. 15–43). Boca Raton, FL: CRC Press, Taylor & Francis.

Cushen, B., Sulaiman, I., Greene, G., MacHale, E., Mokoka, M., Reilly, R. B., . . . Costello, R. W. (2018). The clinical impact of different adherence behaviors in patients with severe chronic obstructive pulmonary disease. *American Journal of Respiratory and Critical Care Medicine, 197*, 1630–1633. http://dx.doi.org/10.1164/rccm.201712-2469LE

Custodio, L. M. (1998). Blowing soap bubbles: Teaching pursed-lip breathing. *Chest, 114*, 1224. http://dx.doi.org/10.1378/chest.114.4.1224

Cystic Fibrosis Foundation. (n.d.-a). *About cystic fibrosis*. Retrieved from http://www.cff.org/What-is-CF/About-Cystic-Fibrosis/

Cystic Fibrosis Foundation. (n.d.-b). *Sweat test*. Retrieved from http://www.cff.org/What-is-CF/Testing/Sweat-Test/

Del Giacco, S. R., Cappai, A., Gambula, L., Cabras, S., Perra, S., Manconi, P. E., . . . Pinna, F. (2016). The asthma-anxiety connection. *Respiratory Medicine, 120*, 44–53. http://dx.doi.org/10.1016/j.rmed.2016.09.014

de Miranda, S., Pochard, F., Chaize, M., Megarbane, B., Cuvelier, A., Bele, N., . . . Azoulay, E. (2011). Postintensive care unit psychological burden in patients with chronic obstructive pulmonary disease and informal caregivers: A multicenter study. *Critical Care Medicine, 39*, 112–118. http://dx.doi.org/10.1097/CCM.0b013e3181feb824

De Peuter, S., Janssens, T., Van Diest, I., Stans, L., Troosters, T., Decramer, M., . . . Vlaeyen, J. W. (2011). Dyspnea-related anxiety: The Dutch version of the Breathlessness Beliefs Questionnaire. *Chronic Respiratory Disease, 8,* 11–19. http://dx.doi.org/10.1177/1479972310383592

DeVito, A. J. (1990). Dyspnea during hospitalizations for acute phase of illness as recalled by patients with chronic obstructive pulmonary disease. *Heart & Lung, 19,* 186–191.

DeVries, R., Kriebel, D., & Sama, S. (2017). Outdoor air pollution and COPD-related emergency department visits, hospital admissions, and mortality: A meta-analysis. *COPD, 14,* 113–121. http://dx.doi.org/10.1080/15412555.2016.1216956

Di Marco, F., Verga, M., Reggente, M., Maria Casanova, F., Santus, P., Blasi, F., . . . Centanni, S. (2006). Anxiety and depression in COPD patients: The roles of gender and disease severity. *Respiratory Medicine, 100,* 1767–1774. http://dx.doi.org/10.1016/j.rmed.2006.01.026

DiMatteo, M. R. (2004a). Social support and patient adherence to medical treatment: A meta-analysis. *Health Psychology, 23,* 207–218. http://dx.doi.org/10.1037/0278-6133.23.2.207

DiMatteo, M. R. (2004b). Variations in patients' adherence to medical recommendations: A quantitative review of 50 years of research. *Medical Care, 42,* 200–209. http://dx.doi.org/10.1097/01.mlr.0000114908.90348.f9

DiTomasso, R. A., Cahn, S. C., Panichelli-Mindel, S. M., & McFillin, R. K. (2013). *Specialty competencies in clinical psychology.* New York, NY: Oxford University Press.

Dobmeyer, A. C. (2018). *Psychological treatment of medical patients in integrated primary care.* Washington, DC: American Psychological Association. http://dx.doi.org/10.1037/0000051-000

Dobmeyer, A. C., & Rowan, A. B. (2014). Core competencies for psychologists: How to succeed in medical settings. In C. M. Hunter, C. L. Hunter, & R. Kessler (Eds.), *Handbook of clinical psychology in medical settings* (pp. 77–98). New York, NY: Springer Science + Business Media.

Doe, S. (2017). Respiratory investigations. In V. Gibson & D. Waters (Eds.), *Respiratory care* (pp. 33–43). Boca Raton, FL: CRC Press/Taylor & Francis.

Donner, C. F., Amaducci, S., Bacci, E., Baldacci, S., Bartoli, M. L., Beghi, G. M., . . . Yu Hui Xin, S. (2018). Inhalation therapy in the next decade: Determinants of adherence to treatment in asthma and COPD. *Archivio Monaldi per le Malattie del Torace, 88,* 886. http://dx.doi.org/10.4081/monaldi.2018.886

Douaihy, A., Stowell, K. R., Park, T. W., & Daley, D. C. (2007). Relapse prevention: Clinical strategies for substance use disorders. In K. Witkiewitz & G. A. Marlatt (Eds.), *Therapist's guide to evidence-based relapse prevention* (pp. 37–71). Amsterdam, Netherlands: Elsevier Academic Press. http://dx.doi.org/10.1016/B978-012369429-4/50033-1

Duarte-de-Araújo, A., Teixeira, P., Hespanhol, V., & Correia-de-Sousa, J. (2018). COPD: Understanding patients' adherence to inhaled medications.

International Journal of Chronic Obstructive Pulmonary Disease, 13, 2767–2773. http://dx.doi.org/10.2147/COPD.S160982

Dunbar-Jacob, J., Gemmell, L. A., & Schlenk, E. A. (2009). Predictors of patient adherence: Patient characteristics. In S. A. Shumaker, J. K. Ockene, & K. A. Riekert (Eds.), *The handbook of health behavior change* (3rd ed., pp. 398–410). New York, NY: Springer. Retrieved from http://search.proquest.com/docview/621662454?accountid=14552

Dunbar-Jacob, J., Schlenk, E., & McCall, M. (2012). *Patient adherence to treatment regimen.* New York, NY: Psychology Press.

Dwyer, M. L., Deshields, T. L., & Nanna, S. K. (2012). Death is a part of life: Considerations for the natural death of a therapy patient. *Professional Psychology: Research and Practice, 43,* 123–129.

Eakin, E. G., Resnikoff, P. M., Prewitt, L. M., Ries, A. L., & Kaplan, R. M. (1998). Validation of a new dyspnea measure: The UCSD Shortness of Breath Questionnaire. University of California, San Diego. *Chest, 113,* 619–624. http://dx.doi.org/10.1378/chest.113.3.619

Ek, K., Ternestedt, B. M., Andershed, B., & Sahlberg-Blom, E. (2011). Shifting life rhythms: Couples' stories about living together when one spouse has advanced chronic obstructive pulmonary disease. *Journal of Palliative Care, 27,* 189–197. http://dx.doi.org/10.1177/082585971102700302

Ekenga, C. C., & Friedman-Jiménez, G. (2011). Epidemiology of respiratory health outcomes among World Trade Center disaster workers: Review of the literature 10 years after the September 11, 2001 terrorist attacks. *Disaster Medicine and Public Health Preparedness, 5,* S189–S196. http://dx.doi.org/10.1001/dmp.2011.58

Federman, A. D., Wolf, M. S., Sofianou, A., Martynenko, M., O'Connor, R., Halm, E. A., . . . Wisnivesky, J. P. (2014). Self-management behaviors in older adults with asthma: Associations with health literacy. *Journal of the American Geriatrics Society, 62,* 872–879. http://dx.doi.org/10.1111/jgs.12797

Figueiredo, D., Gabriel, R., Jácome, C., Cruz, J., & Marques, A. (2014). Caring for relatives with chronic obstructive pulmonary disease: How does the disease severity impact on family carers? *Aging & Mental Health, 18,* 385–393. http://dx.doi.org/10.1080/13607863.2013.837146

Figueiredo, D., Gabriel, R., Jácome, C., & Marques, A. (2014). Caring for people with early and advanced chronic obstructive pulmonary disease: How do family carers cope? *Journal of Clinical Nursing, 23,* 211–220. http://dx.doi.org/10.1111/jocn.12363

Fischer, W., Brandstetter, S., Brandl, M., Finger, T., Böhmer, M. M., Pfeifer, M., & Apfelbacher, C. (2018). Specific, but not general beliefs about medicines are associated with medication adherence in patients with COPD, but not asthma: Cohort study in a population of people with chronic pulmonary disease. *Journal of Psychosomatic Research, 107,* 46–52. http://dx.doi.org/10.1016/j.jpsychores.2018.02.004

Fishwick, D., Sen, D., Barber, C., Bradshaw, L., Robinson, E., Sumner, J., & the COPD Standard Collaboration Group. (2015). Occupational chronic obstructive pulmonary disease: A standard of care. *Occupational Medicine, 65,* 270–282. http://dx.doi.org/10.1093/occmed/kqv019

Flewelling, K. D., Sellers, D. E., Sawicki, G. S., Robinson, W. M., & Dill, E. J. (2019). Social support is associated with fewer reported symptoms and decreased treatment burden in adults with cystic fibrosis. *Journal of Cystic Fibrosis,* http://dx.doi.org/10.1016/j.jcf.2019.01.013

Foggo, B. (2017). Smoking cessation. In V. Gibson & D. Waters (Eds.), *Respiratory care* (pp. 223–233). Boca Raton, FL: CRC Press/Taylor & Francis.

Folstein, M. F., Folstein, S. E., & McHugh, P. R. (1975). "Mini-mental state": A practical method for grading the cognitive state of patients for the clinician. *Journal of Psychiatric Research, 12,* 189–198. http://dx.doi.org/10.1016/0022-3956(75)90026-6

Fontana, L., Lee, S. J., Capitanelli, I., Re, A., Maniscalco, M., Mauriello, M. C., & Iavicoli, I. (2017). Chronic obstructive pulmonary disease in farmers: A systematic review. *Journal of Occupational and Environmental Medicine, 59,* 775–788. http://dx.doi.org/10.1097/JOM.0000000000001072

Food and Drug Administration. (2018). Hookah tobacco. Retrieved from https://www.fda.gov/tobacco-products/products-ingredients-components/hookah-tobacco-shisha-or-waterpipe-tobacco#stats

Ford, E. S., & Wheaton, A. G. (2015). Trends in outpatient visits with benzodiazepines among US adults with and without bronchitis or chronic obstructive pulmonary disease from 1999 to 2010. *COPD, 12,* 649–657.

Foreman, M. G., Zhang, L., Murphy, J., Hansel, N. N., Make, B., Hokanson, J. E., . . . the COPDGene Investigators. (2011). Early-onset chronic obstructive pulmonary disease is associated with female sex, maternal factors, and African American race in the COPD Gene Study. *American Journal of Respiratory and Critical Care Medicine, 184,* 414–420. http://dx.doi.org/10.1164/rccm.201011-1928OC

French, C. T., Irwin, R. S., Fletcher, K. E., & Adams, T. M. (2002). Evaluation of a cough-specific quality-of-life questionnaire. *Chest, 121,* 1123–1131. http://dx.doi.org/10.1378/chest.121.4.1123

Gabriel, R., Figueiredo, D., Jácome, C., Cruz, J., & Marques, A. (2014). Day-to-day living with severe chronic obstructive pulmonary disease: Towards a family-based approach to the illness impacts. *Psychology & Health, 29,* 967–983. http://dx.doi.org/10.1080/08870446.2014.902458

Galvin, W. F. (2016). Patient education. In D. R. Hess, N. R. MacIntyre, W. F. Galvin, & S. C. Mishoe (Eds.), *Respiratory care: Principles and practice* (3rd ed., pp. 707–746). Burlington, MA: Jones & Bartlett Learning.

Gauthier, A., Bernard, S., Bernard, E., Simard, S., Maltais, F., & Lacasse, Y. (2019). Adherence to long-term oxygen therapy in patients with chronic obstructive pulmonary disease. *Chronic Respiratory Disease, 16.* http://dx.doi.org/10.1177/1479972318767724

GBD 2015 Chronic Respiratory Disease Collaborators. (2017). Global, regional, and national deaths, prevalence, disability-adjusted life years, and years lived with disability for chronic obstructive pulmonary disease and asthma, 1990–2015: A systematic analysis for the global burden of disease study 2015. *The Lancet: Respiratory Medicine, 5,* 691–706.

George, J., Kong, D. C., Thoman, R., & Stewart, K. (2005). Factors associated with medication nonadherence in patients with COPD. *Chest, 128,* 3198–3204. http://dx.doi.org/10.1378/chest.128.5.3198

George, M. (2018). Adherence in asthma and COPD: New strategies for an old problem. *Respiratory Care, 63,* 818–831. http://dx.doi.org/10.4187/respcare.05905

Gerke, A. K., Judson, M. A., Cozier, Y. C., Culver, D. A., & Koth, L. L. (2017). Disease burden and variability in sarcoidosis. *Annals of the American Thoracic Society, 14,* S421–S428. http://dx.doi.org/10.1513/AnnalsATS.201707-564OT

Gibson, V., & Waters, D. (2017). *Respiratory care.* Boca Raton, FL: CRC Press/Taylor & Francis.

Glanville, A. R. (Ed.). (2019). *Essentials in lung transplantation.* Cham, Switzerland: Springer International. http://dx.doi.org/10.1007/978-3-319-90933-2

Global Initiative for Asthma. (2018). *Global strategy for asthma management and prevention.* Retrieved from http://www.ginasthma.org

Global Initiative for Chronic Obstructive Lung Disease (GOLD). (2018). *Global strategy for the diagnosis, management, and prevention of chronic obstructive pulmonary disease.* Retrieved from http://www.goldcopd.org

Goessl, V. C., Curtiss, J. E., & Hofmann, S. G. (2017). The effect of heart rate variability biofeedback training on stress and anxiety: A meta-analysis. *Psychological Medicine, 47,* 2578–2586. http://dx.doi.org/10.1017/S0033291717001003

Gold, L. S., Yeung, K., Smith, N., Allen-Ramey, F. C., Nathan, R. A., & Sullivan, S. D. (2013). Asthma control, cost and race: Results from a national survey. *The Journal of Asthma, 50,* 783–790. http://dx.doi.org/10.3109/02770903.2013.795589

Gratziou, Ch., Florou, A., Ischaki, E., Eleftheriou, K., Sachlas, A., Bersimis, S., & Zakynthinos, S. (2014). Smoking cessation effectiveness in smokers with COPD and asthma under real life conditions. *Respiratory Medicine, 108,* 577–583. http://dx.doi.org/10.1016/j.rmed.2014.01.007

Green, J. P., & Lynn, S. J. (2019). *Cognitive-behavioral therapy, mindfulness, and hypnosis for smoking cessation.* Hoboken, NJ: Wiley Blackwell.

Guarnieri, M., & Balmes, J. R. (2014). Outdoor air pollution and asthma. *The Lancet, 383,* 1581–1592. http://dx.doi.org/10.1016/S0140-6736(14)60617-6

Guyatt, G. H., Berman, L. B., Townsend, M., Pugsley, S. O., & Chambers, L. W. (1987). A measure of quality of life for clinical trials in chronic lung disease. *Thorax, 42,* 773–778. http://dx.doi.org/10.1136/thx.42.10.773

Hall, S., Legault, A., & Côté, J. (2010). Dying means suffocating: Perceptions of people living with severe COPD facing the end of life. *International Journal of Palliative Nursing, 16*, 451–457. http://dx.doi.org/10.12968/ijpn.2010.16.9.78640

Han, B., Yan, B., Zhang, J., Zhao, N., Sun, J., Li, C., . . . Chen, J. (2014). The influence of the social support on symptoms of anxiety and depression among patients with silicosis. *The Scientific World Journal, 2014.* http://dx.doi.org/10.1155/2014/724804

Hanson, S. L., Kerkhoff, T. R., & Bush, S. S. (2005). *Health care ethics for psychologists: A casebook.* Washington, DC: American Psychological Association. http://dx.doi.org/10.1037/10845-000

Hartmann-Boyce, J., Chepkin, S. C., Ye, W., Bullen, C., & Lancaster, T. (2018). Nicotine replacement therapy versus control for smoking cessation. *Cochrane Database of Systematic Reviews, 5.* http://dx.doi.org/10.1002/14651858.CD000146.pub5

Hartmann-Boyce, J., McRobbie, H., Bullen, C., Begh, R., Stead, L. F., & Hajek, P. (2016). Electronic cigarettes for smoking cessation. *Cochrane Database of Systematic Reviews, 9.* http://dx.doi.org/10.1002/14651858.CD010216.pub3

Harzheim, D., Klose, H., Pinado, F. P., Ehlken, N., Nagel, C., Fischer, C., . . . Guth, S. (2013). Anxiety and depression disorders in patients with pulmonary arterial hypertension and chronic thromboembolic pulmonary hypertension. *Respiratory Research, 14*, 104. http://dx.doi.org/10.1186/1465-9921-14-104

Haynes, J. (2016). Pulmonary function testing. In D. R. Hess, N. R. MacIntyre, W. F. Galvin, & S. C. Mishoe (Eds.), *Respiratory care: Principles and practice* (3rd ed., pp. 144–170). Burlington, MA: Jones and Bartlett Learning.

Health Grades. (2014). *Prevalence and incidence of sarcoidosis.* Retrieved from https://www.rightdiagnosis.com/s/sarcoidosis/prevalence.htm

Henneberger, P. K., Redlich, C. A., Callahan, D. B., Harber, P., Lemière, C., Martin, J., . . . Torén, K. (2011). An official American Thoracic Society statement: Work-exacerbated asthma. *American Journal of Respiratory and Critical Care Medicine, 184*, 368–378. http://dx.doi.org/10.1164/rccm.812011ST

Hernández Zenteno, R. J., Lara, D. F., Venegas, A. R., Sansores, R. H., Pineda, J. R., Trujillo, F. F., . . . Cazzola, M. (2018). Varenicline for long term smoking cessation in patients with COPD. *Pulmonary Pharmacology & Therapeutics, 53*, 116–120. http://dx.doi.org/10.1016/j.pupt.2018.11.001

Heslop-Marshall, K. (2017). Cognitive behavioural therapy for respiratory conditions. In V. Gibson & D. Waters (Eds.), *Respiratory care* (pp. 247–255). Boca Raton, FL: CRC Press.

Heyland, D. K., Dodek, P., Rocker, G., Groll, D., Gafni, A., Pichora, D., . . . Lam, M. (2006). What matters most in end-of-life care: Perceptions of seriously ill patients and their family members. *Canadian Medical Association Journal, 174*, 627–633.

Holm, K. E., Bowler, R. P., Make, B. J., & Wamboldt, F. S. (2009). Family relationship quality is associated with psychological distress, dyspnea, and quality of life in COPD. *COPD, 6*, 359–368. http://dx.doi.org/10.1080/15412550903143919

Holm, K. E., LaChance, H. R., Bowler, R. P., Make, B. J., & Wamboldt, F. S. (2010). Family factors are associated with psychological distress and smoking status in chronic obstructive pulmonary disease. *General Hospital Psychiatry, 32*, 492–498.

Holt-Lunstad, J. (2018). Why social relationships are important for physical health: A systems approach to understanding and modifying risk and protection. *Annual Review of Psychology, 69*, 437–458. http://dx.doi.org/10.1146/annurev-psych-122216-011902

Horvat, N., Locatelli, I., Kos, M., & Janeûic, A. (2018). Medication adherence and health-related quality of life among patients with chronic obstructive pulmonary disease. *Acta Pharmaceutica, 68*, 117–125. http://dx.doi.org/10.2478/acph-2018-0006

Hoyt, M. A., & Stanton, A. L. (2012). Adjustment to chronic illness. In A. Baum, T. A. Revenson, & J. Singer (Eds.), *Handbook of health psychology* (2nd ed., pp. 219–246). New York, NY: Psychology Press.

Humenberger, M., Horner, A., Labek, A., Kaiser, B., Frechinger, R., Brock, C., . . . Lamprecht, B. (2018). Adherence to inhaled therapy and its impact on chronic obstructive pulmonary disease (COPD). *BMC Pulmonary Medicine, 18*, 163. http://dx.doi.org/10.1186/s12890-018-0724-3

Hunter, C. L., Goodie, J. L., Oordt, M. S., & Dobmeyer, A. C. (2017). *Integrated behavioral health in primary care* (2nd ed.). Washington, DC: American Psychological Association.

Hyland, M. E., Halpin, D. M., Blake, S., Seamark, C., Pinnuck, M., Ward, D., . . . Seamark, D. (2016). Preference for different relaxation techniques by COPD patients: Comparison between six techniques. *International Journal of Chronic Obstructive Pulmonary Disease, 11*, 2315–2319. http://dx.doi.org/10.2147/COPD.S113108

Ingebrigtsen, T. S., Marott, J. L., Nordestgaard, B. G., Lange, P., Hallas, J., Dahl, M., & Vestbo, J. (2015). Low use and adherence to maintenance medication in chronic obstructive pulmonary disease in the general population. *Journal of General Internal Medicine, 30*, 51–59. http://dx.doi.org/10.1007/s11606-014-3029-0

Ingersoll, K. S., & Cohen, J. (2008). The impact of medication regimen factors on adherence to chronic treatment: A review of literature. *Journal of Behavioral Medicine, 31*, 213–224. http://dx.doi.org/10.1007/s10865-007-9147-y

Institute of Medicine. (2004). *Health literacy: A prescription to end confusion.* Washington, DC: The National Academies Press. http://dx.doi.org/10.17226/10883

Ireland, J., & Wilsher, M. (2010). Perceptions and beliefs in sarcoidosis. *Sarcoidosis, Vasculitis, and Diffuse Lung Diseases, 27*, 36–42. Retrieved from https://www.mattioli1885journals.com/index.php/sarcoidosis/article/view/2565

Jácome, C., Figueiredo, D., Gabriel, R., Cruz, J., & Marques, A. (2014). Predicting anxiety and depression among family carers of people with chronic obstructive pulmonary disease. *International Psychogeriatrics, 26*, 1191–1199.

Jenkins, C. R., Chapman, K. R., Donohue, J. F., Roche, N., Tsiligianni, I., & Han, M. K. (2017). Improving the management of COPD in women. *Chest, 151,* 686–696. http://dx.doi.org/10.1016/j.chest.2016.10.031

Jeyashree, K., Kathirvel, S., Shewade, H. D., Kaur, H., & Goel, S. (2016). Smoking cessation interventions for pulmonary tuberculosis treatment outcomes. *The Cochrane Database of Systematic Reviews, 1.* http://dx.doi.org/10.1002/14651858.CD011125.pub2

Jiménez-Ruiz, C. A., Andreas, S., Lewis, K. E., Tonnesen, P., van Schayck, C. P., Hajek, P., . . . Gratziou, C. (2015). Statement on smoking cessation in COPD and other pulmonary diseases and in smokers with comorbidities who find it difficult to quit. *The European Respiratory Journal, 46,* 61–79. http://dx.doi.org/10.1183/09031936.00092614

Johns, M. W. (1991). A new method for measuring daytime sleepiness: The Epworth sleepiness scale. *Sleep, 14,* 540–545. http://dx.doi.org/10.1093/sleep/14.6.540

Jones, K. (2017). *Respiratory disorders sourcebook* (4th ed.). Detroit, MI: Omnigraphics.

Jordan, H. T., Osahan, S., Li, J., Stein, C. R., Friedman, S. M., Brackbill, R. M., . . . Farfel, M. R. (2019). Persistent mental and physical health impact of exposure to the September 11, 2001 World Trade Center terrorist attacks. *Environmental Health: A Global Access Science Source, 18,* 12. http://dx.doi.org/10.1186/s12940-019-0449-7

Judson, M. A., Morgenthau, A. S., & Baughman, R. P. (2016). Sarcoidosis. In V. C. Broaddus, R. J. Mason, J. D. Ernst, T. E. King Jr., S. C. Lazarus, J. F. Murray, . . . M. B. Gotway (Eds.), *Murray and Nadel's textbook of respiratory medicine* (6th ed., pp. 1188–1206.e7). Philadelphia, PA: Elsevier. http://dx.doi.org/10.1016/B978-1-4557-3383-5.00066-X

Juniper, E. F., Guyatt, G. H., Epstein, R. S., Ferrie, P. J., Jaeschke, R., & Hiller, T. K. (1992). Evaluation of impairment of health related quality of life in asthma: Development of a questionnaire for use in clinical trials. *Thorax, 47,* 76–83. http://dx.doi.org/10.1136/thx.47.2.76

Kamil, F., Pinzon, I., & Foreman, M. G. (2013). Sex and race factors in early-onset COPD. *Current Opinion in Pulmonary Medicine, 19,* 140–144. http://dx.doi.org/10.1097/MCP.0b013e32835d903b

Karel, M. J. (2007). Culture and medical decision making. In S. H. Qualls & M. A. Smyer (Eds.), *Changes in decision-making capacity in older adults: Assessment and intervention* (pp. 145–175). Hoboken, NJ: John Wiley & Sons.

Kasper, D. L., Fauci, A. S., Hauser, S. L., Longo, D. L., Jameson, J., & Loscalzo, J. (Eds.). (2016). *Harrison's manual of medicine* (19th ed.). New York, NY: McGraw-Hill.

Katon, W., Von Korff, M., Lin, E., & Simon, G. (2001). Rethinking practitioner roles in chronic illness: The specialist, primary care physician, and the practice nurse. *General Hospital Psychiatry, 23,* 138–144. http://psycnet.apa.org/doi/10.1016/S0163-8343(01)00136-0

Kearney, G. D., Xu, X., Hight, A., & Arcury, T. A. (2013). Case study. Behavior and perception of using safety gear among commercial landscapers: A pilot study. *Journal of Occupational and Environmental Hygiene, 10,* D79–D85. http://dx.doi.org/10.1080/15459624.2013.794381

Kenna, H. A., Poon, A. W., de los Angeles, C. P., & Koran, L. M. (2011). Psychiatric complications of treatment with corticosteroids: Review with case report. *Psychiatry and Clinical Neurosciences, 65,* 549–560. http://dx.doi.org/10.1111/j.1440-1819.2011.02260.x

Kew, K. M., Nashed, M., Dulay, V., & Yorke, J. (2016). Cognitive behavioural therapy (CBT) for adults and adolescents with asthma. *Cochrane Database of Systematic Reviews, 9,* CD011818. http://dx.doi.org/10.1002/14651858. CD011818.pub2

Kirkpatrick, d., & Dransfield, M. T. (2009). Racial and sex differences in chronic obstructive pulmonary disease susceptibility, diagnosis, and treatment. *Current Opinion in Pulmonary Medicine, 15,* 100–104. http://dx.doi.org/10.1097/MCP.0b013e3283232825

Knoll, N., Scholz, U., & Ditzen, B. (2019). Social support, family processes, and health. In T. A. Revenson & R. A. R. Gurung (Eds.), *Handbook of health psychology* (pp. 279–289). New York, NY: Routledge/Taylor & Francis.

Kohansal, R., Martinez-Camblor, P., Agustí, A., Buist, A. S., Mannino, D. M., & Soriano, J. B. (2009). The natural history of chronic airflow obstruction revisited: An analysis of the Framingham offspring cohort. *American Journal of Respiratory and Critical Care Medicine, 180,* 3–10. http://dx.doi.org/10.1164/rccm.200901-0047OC

Kohler, C. L., Fish, L., & Greene, P. G. (2002). The relationship of perceived self-efficacy to quality of life in chronic obstructive pulmonary disease. *Health Psychology, 21,* 610–614. http://dx.doi.org/10.1037/0278-6133.21.6.610

Kohli, P. (2016). Chronic obstructive pulmonary disease. In D. R. Hess, N. R. MacIntyre, W. F. Galvin, & S. C. Mishoe (Eds.), *Respiratory care: Principles and practice* (3rd ed., pp. 801–830). Burlington, MA: Jones & Bartlett Learning.

Kolla, B. P., Foroughi, M., Saeidifard, F., Chakravorty, S., Wang, Z., & Mansukhani, M. P. (2018). The impact of alcohol on breathing parameters during sleep: A systematic review and meta-analysis. *Sleep Medicine Reviews, 42,* 59–67. http://dx.doi.org/10.1016/j.smrv.2018.05.007

Kroenke, K., Spitzer, R. L., & Williams, J. B. (2001). The PHQ-9: Validity of a brief depression severity measure. *Journal of General Internal Medicine, 16,* 606–613. http://dx.doi.org/10.1046/j.1525-1497.2001.016009606.x

Kübler-Ross, E. (1969). *On death and dying.* New York, NY: Macmillan.

Kunik, M. E., Roundy, K., Veazey, C., Souchek, J., Richardson, P., Wray, N. P., & Stanley, M. A. (2005). Surprisingly high prevalence of anxiety and depression in chronic breathing disorders. *Chest, 127,* 1205–1211. http://dx.doi.org/10.1016/S0012-3692(15)34468-8

Kynyk, J. A., Mastronarde, J. G., & McCallister, J. W. (2011). Asthma, the sex difference. *Current Opinion in Pulmonary Medicine, 17*, 6–11. http://dx.doi.org/10.1097/MCP.0b013e3283410038

Labor, S., Labor, M., Jurić, I., & Vuksić, Z. (2012). The prevalence and pulmonary consequences of anxiety and depressive disorders in patients with asthma. *Collegium Antropologicum, 36*, 473–481.

Labott, S. M. (2019). *Health psychology consultation in the inpatient medical setting*. Washington, DC: American Psychological Association. http://dx.doi.org/10.1037/0000108-000

Landsberg, J. W. (2018). *Manual for pulmonary and critical care medicine*. Philadelphia, PA: Elsevier.

Lazarus, R. S., & Folkman, S. (1984). *Stress, appraisal, and coping*. New York, NY: Springer.

Leader, D. (2019). *The link between alcohol and COPD: How drinking may worsen your condition*. Retrieved from http://www.verywellhealth.com/copd-and-alcohol-914949

Lee, S. D., Bender, D. E., Ruiz, R. E., & Cho, Y. I. (2006). Development of an easy-to-use Spanish health literacy test. *Health Services Research, 41*, 1392–1412.

Lee, Y. J., Choi, S. M., Lee, Y. J., Cho, Y. J., Yoon, H. I., Lee, J. H., . . . Park, J. S. (2017). Clinical impact of depression and anxiety in patients with idiopathic pulmonary fibrosis. *PLoS One, 12*, e0184300. http://dx.doi.org/10.1371/journal.pone.0184300

Leo, R. J. (1999). Competency and the capacity to make treatment decisions: A primer for primary care physicians. *Primary Care Companion to the Journal of Clinical Psychiatry, 1*, 131–141. http://dx.doi.org/10.4088/PCC.v01n0501

Lewinsohn, P. M., & Graf, M. (1973). Pleasant activities and depression. *Journal of Consulting and Clinical Psychology, 41*, 261–268.

Lindqvist, G., & Hallberg, L. R-M. (2010). "Feelings of guilt due to self-inflicted disease": A grounded theory of suffering from chronic obstructive pulmonary disease (COPD). *Journal of Health Psychology, 15*, 456–466. http://dx.doi.org/10.1177/1359105309353646

Liptzin, B., & Levkoff, S. E. (1992). An empirical study of delirium subtypes. *The British Journal of Psychiatry, 161*, 843–845. http://dx.doi.org/10.1192/bjp.161.6.843

Lowe, B., Grafe, K., Ufer, C., Kroenke, K., Grunig, E., Herzog, W., & Borst, M. M. (2004). Anxiety and depression in patients with pulmonary hypertension. *Psychosomatic Medicine, 66*, 831–836. http://dx.doi.org/10.1097/01.psy.0000145593.37594.39

Lowery, E. M., Yong, M., Cohen, A., Joyce, C., & Kovacs, E. J. (2018). Recent alcohol use prolongs hospital length of stay following lung transplant. *Clinical Transplantation, 32*, e13250. http://dx.doi.org/10.1111/ctr.13250

Lowey, S. E., Norton, S. A., Quinn, J. R., & Quill, T. E. (2013). Living with advanced heart failure or COPD: Experiences and goals of individuals nearing the end of life. *Research in Nursing & Health, 36,* 349–358. http://dx.doi.org/10.1002/nur.21546

Lucas, D., Lodde, B., Jepsen, J. R., Dewitte, J. D., & Jegaden, D. (2016). Occupational asthma in maritime environments: An update. *International Maritime Health, 67,* 144–152. http://dx.doi.org/10.5603/IMH.2016.0027

MacIntyre, N. R., & Crouch, R. H. (2016). Pulmonary rehabilitation. In D. R. Hess, N. R. MacIntyre, W. F. Galvin, & S. C. Mishoe (Eds.), *Respiratory care: Principles and practice* (3rd ed., pp. 594–605). Burlington, MA: Jones & Bartlett Learning.

Mamane, A., Baldi, I., Tessier, J. F., Raherison, C., & Bouvier, G. (2015). Occupational exposure to pesticides and respiratory health. *European Respiratory Review, 24,* 306–319. http://dx.doi.org/10.1183/16000617.00006014

Matsuse, H. (2016). Mechanism and management of alcohol-induced asthma. *Nihon Arukoru Yakubutsu Igakkai Zasshi, 51,* 214–220.

Maurer, J., Rebbapragada, V., Borson, S., Goldstein, R., Kunik, M. E., Yohannes, A. M., & Hanania, N. A. (2008). Anxiety and depression in COPD: Current understanding, unanswered questions, and research needs. *Chest, 134,* 43S–56S. http://dx.doi.org/10.1378/chest.08-0342

Mayo Clinic. (n.d.). *Pulmonary fibrosis.* Retrieved from http://www.mayoclinic.org/diseases-conditions/pulmonary-fibrosis/symptoms-causes/syc-20353690

Mayo Clinic. (2016, October 13). *Cystic fibrosis.* Retrieved from http://www.mayoclinic.org/diseases-conditions/cystic-fibrosis/symptoms-causes/syc-20353700

Mayo Clinic. (2017). *Pulmonary hypertension.* Retrieved from http://www.mayoclinic.org/diseases-conditions/pulmonary-hypertension/symptoms-causes/syc-20350697

Mazurek, J. M., & Weissman, D. N. (2016). Occupational respiratory allergic diseases in healthcare workers. *Current Allergy and Asthma Reports, 16,* 77. http://dx.doi.org/10.1007/s11882-016-0657-y

McCathie, H. C., Spence, S. H., & Tate, R. L. (2002). Adjustment to chronic obstructive pulmonary disease: The importance of psychological factors. *The European Respiratory Journal, 19,* 47–53. http://dx.doi.org/10.1183/09031936.02.00240702

McConnaughy, E. A., DiClemente, C. C., Prochaska, J. O., & Velicer, W. F. (1989). Stages of change in psychotherapy: A follow-up report. *Psychotherapy: Theory, Research, Practice, Training, 26,* 494–503.

McEwen, A., Hajek, P., McRobbie, H., & West, R. (2006). *Manual of smoking cessation.* Malden, MA: Blackwell. http://dx.doi.org/10.1002/9780470757864

McLeish, A. C., Farris, S. G., Johnson, A. L., Bernstein, J. A., & Zvolensky, M. J. (2016). Evaluation of smokers with and without asthma in terms of smoking cessation outcome, nicotine withdrawal symptoms, and craving: Findings from a self-guided quit attempt. *Addictive Behaviors, 63,* 149–154. http://dx.doi.org/10.1016/j.addbeh.2016.07.021

McQuaid, E. L. (2018). Barriers to medication adherence in asthma: The importance of culture and context. *Annals of Allergy, Asthma & Immunology, 121,* 37–42. http://dx.doi.org/10.1016/j.anai.2018.03.024

Medscape. (2018). *What is the prevalence of pulmonary arterial hypertension (PAH)?* Retrieved from https://www.medscape.com/answers/303098-93384/what-is-the-prevalence-of-pulmonary-arterial-hypertension-pah

Meier, C., Bodenmann, G., Moergeli, H., & Jenewein, J. (2011). Dyadic coping, quality of life, and psychological distress among chronic obstructive pulmonary disease patients and their partners. *International Journal of Chronic Obstructive Pulmonary Disease, 6,* 583–596. http://dx.doi.org/10.2147/COPD.S24508

Meier, C., Bodenmann, G., Moergeli, H., Peter-Wight, M., Martin, M., Buechi, S., & Jenewein, J. (2012). Dyadic coping among couples with COPD: A pilot study. *Journal of Clinical Psychology in Medical Settings, 19,* 243–254. http://psycnet.apa.org/doi/10.1007/s10880-011-9279-7

Mesquita, C. B., Knaut, C., Caram, L. M. O., Ferrari, R., Bazan, S. G. Z., Godoy, I., & Tanni, S. E. (2018). Impact of adherence to long-term oxygen therapy on patients with COPD and exertional hypoxemia followed for one year. *Jornal Brasileiro De Pneumologia: Publicacao Oficial Da Sociedade Brasileira De Pneumologia e Tisilogia, 44,* 390–397. http://dx.doi.org/10.1590/s1806-37562017000000019

Mi, E., Mi, E., Ewing, G., Mahadeva, R., Gardener, A. C., Holt Butcher, H., . . . Farquhar, M. (2017). Associations between the psychological health of patients and carers in advanced COPD. *International Journal of Chronic Obstructive Pulmonary Disease, 12,* 2813–2821. http://dx.doi.org/10.2147/COPD.S139188

Miccinesi, G., Bianchi, E., Brunelli, C., & Borreani, C. (2012). End-of-life preferences in advanced cancer patients willing to discuss issues surrounding their terminal condition. *European Journal of Cancer Care, 21,* 623–633. http://dx.doi.org/10.1111/j.1365-2354.2012.01347.x

Miller, W. R., & Rollnick, S. (2013). *Motivational interviewing: Helping people change.* New York, NY: Guilford Press.

Millon, T., Antoni, M., Millon, C., Minor, S., & Grossman, S. (2001). Millon Behavioral Medicine Diagnostic (MBMD). Retrieved from https://www.pearsonclinical.com/psychology/products/100000231/millon-behavioral-medicine-diagnostic-mbmd.html

Miravitlles, M., & Ribera, A. (2017). Understanding the impact of symptoms on the burden of COPD. *Respiratory Research, 18,* 67–78. http://dx.doi.org/10.1186/s12931-017-0548-3

Mukundu, L., & Matiti, M. R. (2015). Managing COPD using pulmonary rehabilitation: A literature review. *Nursing Standard, 30,* 38–43. http://dx.doi.org/10.7748/ns.30.14.38.s44

Myers, T. R., & Op't Holt, T. (2016). Asthma. In D. R. Hess, N. R. MacIntyre, W. F. Galvin, & S. C. Mishoe (Eds.), *Respiratory care: Principles and practice* (3rd ed., pp. 766–800). Burlington, MA: Jones & Bartlett Learning.

National Heart, Lung, and Blood Institute. (n.d.). Asthma. Retrieved from https://www.nhlbi.nih.gov/health-topics/asthma

National Institutes of Health, U.S. National Library of Medicine. (2019). *Idiopathic pulmonary fibrosis*. Retrieved from https://ghr.nlm.nih.gov/condition/idiopathic-pulmonary-fibrosis#statistics

National POLST Paradigm. (n.d.). Retrieved from https://www.polst.org

O'Conor, R., Muellers, K., Arvanitis, M., Vicencio, D. P., Wolf, M. S., Wisnivesky, J. P., & Federman, A. D. (2019, November–December). Effects of health literacy and cognitive abilities on COPD self-management behaviors: A prospective cohort study. *Respiratory Medicine, 160.* http://dx.doi.org/10.1016/j.rmed.2019.02.006

Omachi, T. A., Sarkar, U., Yelin, E. H., Blanc, P. D., & Katz, P. P. (2013). Lower health literacy is associated with poorer health status and outcomes in chronic obstructive pulmonary disease. *Journal of General Internal Medicine, 28,* 74–81. http://dx.doi.org/10.1007/s11606-012-2177-3

Ouellette, D. R., & Lavoie, K. L. (2017). Recognition, diagnosis, and treatment of cognitive and psychiatric disorders in patients with COPD. *International Journal of Chronic Obstructive Pulmonary Disease, 12,* 639–650. http://dx.doi.org/10.2147/COPD.S123994

Panagioti, M., Scott, C., Blakemore, A., & Coventry, P. A. (2014). Overview of the prevalence, impact, and management of depression and anxiety in chronic obstructive pulmonary disease. *International Journal of Chronic Obstructive Pulmonary Disease, 9,* 1289–1306. http://dx.doi.org/10.2147/COPD.S72073

Papaioannou, A. I., Tsikrika, S., Bartziokas, K., Karakontaki, F., Kastanakis, E., Diamantea, F., . . . Kostikas, K. (2014). Collateral damage: Depressive symptoms in the partners of COPD patients. *Lung, 192,* 519–524. http://dx.doi.org/10.1007/s00408-014-9595-4

Park, E. R., Gareen, I. F., Japuntich, S., Lennes, I., Hyland, K., DeMello, S., . . . Rigotti, N. A. (2015). Primary care provider-delivered smoking cessation interventions and smoking cessation among participants in the National Lung Screening Trial. *JAMA Internal Medicine, 175,* 1509–1516. http://dx.doi.org/10.1001/jamainternmed.2015.2391

Parry, G. D., Cooper, C. L., Moore, J. M., Yadegarfar, G., Campbell, M. J., Esmonde, L., . . . Hutchcroft, B. J. (2012). Cognitive behavioural intervention for adults with anxiety complications of asthma: Prospective randomised trial. *Respiratory Medicine, 106,* 802–810. http://dx.doi.org/10.1016/j.rmed.2012.02.006

Perret, J. L., Boneveski, B., McDonald, C. F., & Abramson, M. J. (2016). Smoking cessation strategies for patients with asthma: Improving patient outcomes.

Journal of Asthma and Allergy, 9, 117–128. http://dx.doi.org/10.2147/JAA.S85615

Plaza, V., López-Viña, A., Entrenas, L. M., Fernández-Rodríguez, C., Melero, C., Pérez-Llano, L., . . . Cosio, B. G. (2016). Differences in adherence and non-adherence behaviour patterns to inhaler devices between COPD and asthma patients. *COPD, 13,* 547–554. http://dx.doi.org/10.3109/15412555.2015.1118449

Politis, A., Ioannidis, V., Gourgoulianis, K. I., Daniil, Z., & Hatzoglou, C. (2018). Effects of varenicline therapy in combination with advanced behavioral support on smoking cessation and quality of life in inpatients with acute exacerbation of COPD, bronchial asthma, or community-acquired pneumonia: A prospective, open-label, preference-based, 52-week, follow-up trial. *Chronic Respiratory Disease, 15,* 146–156. http://dx.doi.org/10.1177/1479972317740128

Pollok, J., van Agteren, J. E., & Carson-Chahhoud, K. V. (2018). Pharmacological interventions for the treatment of depression in chronic obstructive pulmonary disease. *Cochrane Database of Systematic Reviews, 12,* CD012346. http://dx.doi.org/10.1002/14651858.CD012346.pub2

Popa-Velea, O., & Purcarea, V. L. (2014). Psychological factors mediating health-related quality of life in COPD. *Journal of Medicine and Life, 7,* 100–103.

Pope, T. M., & Hexum, M. (2012). Legal briefing: POLST: Physician orders for life-sustaining treatment. *The Journal of Clinical Ethics, 23,* 353–376.

Powers, M. B., de Kleine, R. A., & Smits, J. A. J. (2017). Core mechanisms of cognitive behavioral therapy for anxiety and depression: A review. *The Psychiatric Clinics of North America, 40,* 611–623. http://dx.doi.org/10.1016/j.psc.2017.08.010

Priestley, L., Green, C., & Abel, Z. (2017). Cystic fibrosis. In V. Gibson & D. Waters (Eds.), *Respiratory care* (pp. 159–168). Boca Raton, FL: CRC Press/Taylor & Francis.

Prochaska, J. O., DiClemente, C. C., & Norcross, J. C. (1992). In search of how people change. Applications to addictive behaviors. *American Psychologist, 47,* 1102–1114. http://dx.doi.org/10.1037/0003-066X.47.9.1102

Puente-Maestu, L., Calle, M., Rodríguez-Hermosa, J. L., Campuzano, A., de Miguel Díez, J., Álvarez-Sala, J. L., . . . Lee, S. Y. (2016). Health literacy and health outcomes in chronic obstructive pulmonary disease. *Respiratory Medicine, 115,* 78–82. http://dx.doi.org/10.1016/j.rmed.2016.04.016

Puhan, M. A., Gimeno-Santos, E., Cates, C. J., & Troosters, T. (2016). Pulmonary rehabilitation following exacerbations of chronic obstructive pulmonary disease. *Cochrane Database of Systematic Reviews, 12,* CD005305. http://dx.doi.org/10.1002/14651858.CD005305.pub4

Pulmonary Fibrosis Foundation. (2019). Causes and symptoms of pulmonary fibrosis. Retrieved from http://www.pulmonaryfibrosis.org/life-with-pf/about-pf

Quinn, V. P., Hollis, J. F., Smith, K. S., Rigotti, N. A., Solberg, L. I., Hu, W., & Stevens, V. J. (2009). Effectiveness of the 5-As tobacco cessation treatments in nine HMOs. *Journal of General Internal Medicine, 24,* 149–154. http://dx.doi.org/10.1007/s11606-008-0865-9

Quittner, A. L., Buu, A., Messer, M. A., Modi, A. C., & Watrous, M. (2005). Development and validation of the Cystic Fibrosis Questionnaire in the United States. *Chest, 128,* 2347–2354. http://dx.doi.org/10.1378/chest.128.4.2347

Quittner, A. L., Goldbeck, L., Abbott, J., Duff, A., Lambrecht, P., Solé, A., . . . Barker, D. (2014). Prevalence of depression and anxiety in patients with cystic fibrosis and parent caregivers: Results of The International Depression Epidemiological Study across nine countries. *Thorax, 69,* 1090–1097. http://dx.doi.org/10.1136/thoraxjnl-2014-205983

Raad, D., Gaddam, S., Schunemann, H. J., Irani, J., Abou Jaoude, P., Honeine, R., & Akl, E. A. (2011). Effects of water-pipe smoking on lung function: A systematic review and meta-analysis. *Chest, 139,* 764–774. http://dx.doi.org/10.1378/chest.10-0991

Raghavan, D., & Jain, R. (2016). Increasing awareness of sex differences in airway diseases. *Respirology, 21,* 449–459. http://dx.doi.org/10.1111/resp.12702

Rainer, J. P., Thompson, C. H., & Lambros, H. (2010). Psychological and psychosocial aspects of the solid organ transplant experience—A practice review. *Psychotherapy: Theory, Research, Practice, Training, 47,* 403–412. http://psycnet.apa.org/doi/10.1037/a0021167

Rajala, K., Lehto, J. T., Saarinen, M., Sutinen, E., Saarto, T., & Myllarniemi, M. (2016). End-of-life care of patients with idiopathic pulmonary fibrosis. *BMC Palliative Care, 15,* 85. http://dx.doi.org/10.1186/s12904-016-0158-8

Reardon, J. Z. (2007). Environmental tobacco smoke: Respiratory and other health effects. *Clinics in Chest Medicine, 28,* 559–573. http://dx.doi.org/10.1016/j.ccm.2007.06.006

Resnicow, K., DiIorio, C., Soet, J. E., Borrelli, B., Hecht, J., & Ernst, D. (2002). Motivational interviewing in health promotion: It sounds like something is changing. *Health Psychology, 21,* 444–451.

Ribeiro, L., & Ind, P. W. (2018). Marijuana and the lung: Hysteria or cause for concern? *Breathe, 14,* 196–205. http://dx.doi.org/10.1183/20734735.020418

Rigotti, N. A. (2013). Smoking cessation in patients with respiratory disease: Existing treatments and future directions. *The Lancet: Respiratory Medicine, 1,* 241–250. http://dx.doi.org/10.1016/S2213-2600(13)70063-8

Rocker, G. M., Dodek, P. M., & Heyland, D. K. (2008). Toward optimal end-of-life care for patients with advanced chronic obstructive pulmonary disease: Insights from a multicentre study. *Canadian Respiratory Journal, 15,* 249–254. http://dx.doi.org/10.1155/2008/369162

Rogliani, P., Ora, J., Puxeddu, E., Matera, M. G., & Cazzola, M. (2017). Adherence to COPD treatment: Myth and reality. *Respiratory Medicine, 129*, 117–123. http://dx.doi.org/10.1016/j.rmed.2017.06.007

Rolnick, S. J., Pawloski, P. A., Hedblom, B. D., Asche, S. E., & Bruzek, R. J. (2013). Patient characteristics associated with medication adherence. *Clinical Medicine & Research, 11*, 54–65. http://dx.doi.org/10.3121/cmr.2013.1113

Rotenberg, B. W., Murariu, D., & Pang, K. P. (2016). Trends in CPAP adherence over twenty years of data collection: A flattened curve. *Head & Neck Surgery, 45*, 43. http://dx.doi.org/10.1186/s40463-016-0156-0

Rowe, S. M., Hoover, W., & Solomon, G. M. (2016). Cystic fibrosis. In V. C. Broaddus, R. J. Mason, J. D. Ernst, T. E. King Jr., S. C. Lazarus, J. F. Murray, . . . M. B. Gotway (Eds.), *Murray & Nadel's textbook of respiratory medicine* (6th ed., pp. 822–852.e17). Pittsburgh, PA: Elsevier. http://dx.doi.org/10.1016/B978-1-4557-3383-5.00047-6

Rzadkiewicz, M., Bråtas, O., & Espnes, G. A. (2016). What else should we know about experiencing COPD? A narrative review in search of patients' psychological burden alleviation. *International Journal of Chronic Obstructive Pulmonary Disease, 11*, 2295–2304. http://dx.doi.org/10.2147/COPD.S109700

Sampaio, M. S., Vieira, W. A., Bernardino, I. M., Herval, A. M., Flores-Mir, C., & Paranhos, L. R. (2019). Chronic obstructive pulmonary disease as a risk factor for suicide: A systematic review and meta-analysis. *Respiratory Medicine, 151*, 11–18. http://dx.doi.org/10.1016/j.rmed.2019.03.018

Sanduzzi, A., Balbo, P., Candoli, P., Catapano, G. A., Contini, P., Mattei, A., . . . Stanziola, A. A. (2014). COPD: Adherence to therapy. *Multidisciplinary Respiratory Medicine, 9*, 60. http://dx.doi.org/10.1186/2049-6958-9-60

Seaman, D. M., Meyer, C. A., & Kanne, J. P. (2015). Occupational and environmental lung disease. *Clinics in Chest Medicine, 36*, 249–268. http://dx.doi.org/10.1016/j.ccm.2015.02.008

Searight, H. R. (1992). Assessing patient competence for medical decision making. *American Family Physician, 45*, 751–759.

Self, T. H., Shah, S. P., March, K. L., & Sands, C. W. (2017). Asthma associated with the use of cocaine, heroin, and marijuana: A review of the evidence. *Journal of Asthma, 54*, 714–722. http://dx.doi.org/10.1080/02770903.2016.1259420

Seneviratne, I. N. S., & Hopkins, P. (2019). Who and when to transplant: What has changed? In A. R. Glanville (Ed.), *Essentials in lung transplantation* (pp. 1–17). Cham, Switzerland: Springer. http://dx.doi.org/10.1007/978-3-319-90933-2_1

Sesé, L., Nunes, H., Cottin, V., Sanyal, S., Didier, M., Carton, Z., . . . Annesi-Maesano, I. (2018). Role of atmospheric pollution on the natural history of idiopathic pulmonary fibrosis. *Thorax, 73*, 145–150. http://dx.doi.org/10.1136/thoraxjnl-2017-209967

Shirley, B. (2006). Hypnosis for smoking cessation. *Australian Journal of Clinical Hypnotherapy and Hypnosis, 27,* 17–22.

Short, K. A., & Ghio, A. J. (2016). Interstitial lung disease. In D. R. Hess, N. R. MacIntyre, W. F. Galvin, & S. C. Mishoe (Eds.), *Respiratory care: Principles and practice* (3rd ed., pp. 831–844). Burlington, MA: Jones & Bartlett Learning.

Simmons, P. (2016). Respiratory assessment. In D. R. Hess, N. R. MacIntyre, W. F. Galvin, & S. C. Mishoe (Eds.), *Respiratory care: Principles and practice* (3rd ed., pp. 2–21). Burlington, MA: Jones & Bartlett Learning.

Simon, G. E. (2002). Evidence review: Efficacy and effectiveness of anti-depressant treatment in primary care. *General Hospital Psychiatry, 24,* 213–224. http://dx.doi.org/10.1016/S0163-8343(02)00198-6

Singh, V. P., Rao, V., Prem, V., Sahoo, R. C., & Keshav, P. K. (2009). Comparison of the effectiveness of music and progressive muscle relaxation for anxiety in COPD—A randomized controlled pilot study. *Chronic Respiratory Disease, 6,* 209–216. http://dx.doi.org/10.1177/1479972309346754

Slok, A. H., Bemelmans, T. C., Kotz, D., van der Molen, T., & Kerstjens, H. A. In't Veen, J. C., . . . van Schayck, O. C. (2016). The Assessment of Burden of COPD (ABC) scale: A reliable and valid questionnaire. *COPD, 13,* 431–438. http://dx.doi.org/10.3109/15412555.2015.1118025

Smith, S. M., Sonego, S., Ketcheson, L., & Larson, J. L. (2014). A review of the effectiveness of psychological interventions used for anxiety and depression in chronic obstructive pulmonary disease. *BMJ Open Respiratory Research, 1,* e000042-2014-000042. http://dx.doi.org/10.1136/bmjresp-2014-000042

Smyth, J. M., Zawadzki, M. J., Santuzzi, A. M., & Filipkowski, K. B. (2014). Examining the effects of perceived social support on momentary mood and symptom reports in asthma and arthritis patients. *Psychology & Health, 29,* 813–831. http://dx.doi.org/10.1080/08870446.2014.889139

Snyder, B., & Cunningham, R. L. (2018). Sex differences in sleep apnea and comorbid neurodegenerative diseases. *Steroids, 133,* 28–33. http://dx.doi.org/10.1016/j.steroids.2017.12.006

Solano, J. P., Gomes, B., & Higginson, I. J. (2006). A comparison of symptom prevalence in far advanced cancer, AIDS, heart disease, chronic obstructive pulmonary disease and renal disease. *Journal of Pain and Symptom Management, 31,* 58–69. http://dx.doi.org/10.1016/j.jpainsymman.2005.06.007

Soones, T. N., Lin, J. L., Wolf, M. S., O'Conor, R., Martynenko, M., Wisnivesky, J. P., & Federman, A. D. (2017). Pathways linking health literacy, health beliefs, and cognition to medication adherence in older adults with asthma. *The Journal of Allergy and Clinical Immunology, 139,* 804–809. http://dx.doi.org/10.1016/j.jaci.2016.05.043

Spitzer, R. L., Kroenke, K., & Williams, J. B. (1999). Validation and utility of a self-report version of PRIME-MD: The PHQ primary care study. *JAMA, 282,* 1737–1744. http://dx.doi.org/10.1001/jama.282.18.1737

Spitzer, R. L., Williams, J. B. W., Kroenke, K. et al. (n.d.). *Patient Health Questionnaire (PHQ) screeners.* https://www.phqscreeners.com/select-screener/

Stave, G. M. (2018). Occupational animal allergy. *Current Allergy and Asthma Reports, 18*, 11. http://dx.doi.org/10.1007/s11882-018-0755-0

Stenton, C. (2017). Occupational lung disease. In V. Gibson & D. Waters (Eds.), *Respiratory care* (pp. 111–122). Boca Raton, FL: CRC Press/Taylor & Francis.

Stoleski, S., Minov, J., Karadzinska-Bislimovska, J., & Mijakoski, D. (2015). Chronic obstructive pulmonary disease in never-smoking dairy farmers. *The Open Respiratory Medicine Journal, 9*, 59–66. http://dx.doi.org/10.2174/1874306401509010059

Strid, J. M., Christiansen, C. F., Olsen, M., & Qin, P. (2014). Hospitalisation for chronic obstructive pulmonary disease and risk of suicide: A population-based case-control study. *British Medical Journal Open.* http://dx.doi.org/10.1136/bmjopen-2014-006363

Strub, R. L., & Black, F. W. (2000). *The mental status examination in neurology* (4th ed.). Philadelphia, PA: F. A. Davis.

Substance Abuse and Mental Health Services Administration. (2019a). *Key substance use and mental health indicators in the United States: Results from the 2018 National Survey on Drug Use and Health* (HHS Publication No. PEP19-5068, NSDUH Series H-54). Rockville, MD: Center for Behavioral Health Statistics and Quality, Substance Abuse and Mental Health Services Administration. Retrieved from https://www.samhsa.gov/data/sites/default/files/cbhsq-reports/NSDUHNationalFindingsReport2018/NSDUHNationalFindingsReport2018.pdf

Substance Abuse and Mental Health Services Administration. (2019b). *Results from the 2018 National Survey on Drug Use and Health: Detailed tables.* Rockville, MD: Center for Behavioral Health Statistics and Quality, Substance Abuse and Mental Health Services Administration. Retrieved from https://www.samhsa.gov/data/

Sussman, L. K. (2004). The role of culture in definitions, interpretations, and management of illness. In U. P. Gielen, J. M. Fish, & J. G. Draguns (Eds.), *Handbook of culture, therapy, and healing* (pp. 37–65). Mahwah, NJ: Lawrence Erlbaum.

Sussman, L. K. (2008). The role of culture in illness interpretation and therapy. In U. P. Gielen, J. G. Draguns, & J. M. Fish (Eds.), *Principles of multicultural counseling and therapy* (pp. 37–70). New York, NY: Routledge/Taylor & Francis Group.

Sutherland, E. R., Sciurba, F. C., Glazer, C. S., & Halpern, S. D. (2012). Clinical year in review III: Asthma, chronic obstructive pulmonary disease, environmental and occupational lung disease, and ethics and end-of-life care. *Proceedings of the American Thoracic Society, 9*, 197–203. http://dx.doi.org/10.1513/pats.201206-032TT

Tan, W. C., Lo, C., Jong, A., Xing, L., Fitzgerald, M. J., Vollmer, W. M., . . . Sin, D. D. (2009). Marijuana and chronic obstructive lung disease: A population-based study. *CMAJ, 180,* 814–820. http://dx.doi.org/10.1503/cmaj.081040

Tan, W. C., & Sin, D. D. (2018). What are the long-term effects of smoked marijuana on lung health? *CMAJ, 190,* E1243–E1244. http://dx.doi.org/10.1503/cmaj.181307

Tashkin, D. P. (2015). Smoking cessation in chronic obstructive pulmonary disease. *Seminars in Respiratory and Critical Care Medicine, 36,* 491–507. http://dx.doi.org/10.1055/s-0035-1555610

Tashkin, D. P. (2018). Marijuana and lung disease. *Chest, 154,* 653–663. http://dx.doi.org/10.1016/j.chest.2018.05.005

Taveira, K. V. M., Kuntze, M. M., Berretta, F., de Souza, B. D. M., Godolfim, L. R., Demathe, T., . . . Porporatti, A. L. (2018). Association between obstructive sleep apnea and alcohol, caffeine and tobacco: A meta-analysis. *Journal of Oral Rehabilitation, 45,* 890–902. http://dx.doi.org/10.1111/joor.12686

Teng, E. L., & Chui, H. C. (1987). The Modified Mini-Mental State (3MS) examination. *The Journal of Clinical Psychiatry, 48,* 314–318.

Tetikkurt, C., Ozdemir, I., Tetikkurt, S., Yilmaz, N., Ertan, T., & Bayar, N. (2011). Anxiety and depression in COPD patients and correlation with sputum and BAL cytology. *Multidisciplinary Respiratory Medicine, 6,* 226–231. http://dx.doi.org/10.1186/2049-6958-6-4-226

Tiemensma, J., Gaab, E., Voorhaar, M., Asijee, G., & Kaptein, A. A. (2016). Illness perceptions and coping determine quality of life in COPD patients. *International Journal of Chronic Obstructive Pulmonary Disease, 11,* 2001–2007. http://dx.doi.org/10.2147/COPD.S109227

Torres-Sánchez, I., Rodríguez-Alzueta, E., Cabrera-Martos, I., López-Torres, I., Moreno-Ramírez, M. P., & Valenza, M. C. (2015). Cognitive impairment in COPD: A systematic review. *Jornal Brasileiro De Pneumologia, 41,* 182–190. http://dx.doi.org/10.1590/S1806-37132015000004424

Trent, S. A., Hasegawa, K., Ramratnam, S. K., Bittner, J. C., & Camargo, C. A., Jr. (2017). Variation in asthma care at hospital discharge by race/ethnicity groups. *The Journal of Asthma,* 1–10. http://dx.doi.org/10.1080/02770903.2017.1378356

Trethewey, S. P., & Walters, G. I. (2018). The role of occupational and environmental exposures in the pathogenesis of idiopathic pulmonary fibrosis: A narrative literature review. *Medicina, 54.* http://dx.doi.org/10.3390/medicina54060108

Trivedi, R. B., Bryson, C. L., Udris, E., & Au, D. H. (2012). The influence of informal caregivers on adherence in COPD patients. *Annals of Behavioral Medicine, 44,* 66–72. http://dx.doi.org/10.1007/s12160-012-9355-8

Trivedi, V., Apala, D. R., & Iyer, V. N. (2017). Occupational asthma: Diagnostic challenges and management dilemmas. *Current Opinion in Pulmonary Medicine, 23,* 177–183. http://dx.doi.org/10.1097/MCP.0000000000000352

Tselebis, A., Bratis, D., Pachi, A., Moussas, G., Karkanias, A., Harikiopoulou, M., . . . Tzanakis, N. (2013). Chronic obstructive pulmonary disease: Sense of coherence and family support versus anxiety and depression. *Psychiatriki, 24,* 109–116.

Tselebis, A., Pachi, A., Ilias, I., Kosmas, E., Bratis, D., Moussas, G., & Tzanakis, N. (2016). Strategies to improve anxiety and depression in patients with COPD: A mental health perspective. *Neuropsychiatric Disease and Treatment, 12,* 297–328. http://dx.doi.org/10.2147/NDT.S79354

Tsiligianni, I., Rodriguez, M. R., Lisspers, K., LeeTan, T., & Infantino, A. (2017). Call to action: Improving primary care for women with COPD. *NPJ Primary Care Respiratory Medicine, 27,* 11. http://dx.doi.org/10.1038/s41533-017-0013-2

Tucker, E., & Stoermer, C. (2017). Pulmonary rehabilitation. In V. Gibson & D. Waters (Eds.), *Respiratory care* (pp. 235–246). Boca Raton, FL: CRC Press/ Taylor & Francis.

Turan, O., Turan, P. A., & Mirici, A. (2017). Parameters affecting inhalation therapy adherence in elderly patients with chronic obstructive lung disease and asthma. *Geriatrics & Gerontology International, 17,* 999–1005. http:// dx.doi.org/10.1111/ggi.12823

U.S. Department of Health and Human Services. (2014). *The health consequences of smoking: 50 years of progress. A report of the surgeon general* [Printed with corrections, January 2014]. Atlanta, GA: U.S. Department of Health and Human Services, Centers for Disease Control and Prevention, National Center for Chronic Disease Prevention and Health Promotion, Office on Smoking and Health.

U.S. Department of Health and Human Services. (2018). *The COPD National Action Plan*. Retrieved from https://www.nhlbi.nih.gov/health-topics/ education-and-awareness/COPD-national-action-plan

U.S. Department of Health and Human Services, Office of Disease Prevention and Health Promotion. (2010). *National action plan to improve health literacy*. Washington, DC: Author. Retrieved from https://health.gov/sites/default/ files/2019-09/Health_Literacy_Action_Plan.pdf

van Boven, J. F., Chavannes, N. H., van der Molen, T., Rutten-van Mölken, M. P., Postma, M. J., & Vegter, S. (2014). Clinical and economic impact of non-adherence in COPD: A systematic review. *Respiratory Medicine, 108,* 103–113. http://dx.doi.org/10.1016/j.rmed.2013.08.044

van Eerd, E. A., van der Meer, R. M., van Schayck, O. C., & Kotz, D. (2016). Smoking cessation for people with chronic obstructive pulmonary disease. *Cochrane Database of Systematic Reviews, CD010744*. http://dx.doi.org/10.1002/ 14651858.CD010744.pub2

Venkat, A., Hasegawa, K., Basior, J. M., Crandall, C., Healy, M., Inboriboon, P. C., . . . Camargo, C. A., Jr. (2015). Race/ethnicity and asthma management among adults presenting to the emergency department. *Respirology, 20,* 994–997. http://dx.doi.org/10.1111/resp.12572

Volpato, E., Banfi, P., Rogers, S. M., & Pagnini, F. (2015). Relaxation techniques for people with chronic obstructive pulmonary disease: A systematic review and a meta-analysis. *Evidence-Based Complementary and Alternative Medicine, 2015,* 1. http://dx.doi.org/10.1155/2015/628365

Volsko, T. A., O'Malley, C., & Rubin, B. K. (2016). Cystic fibrosis. In D. R. Hess, N. R. MacIntyre, W. F. Galvin, & S. C. Mishoe (Eds.), *Respiratory care: Principles and practice* (3rd ed., pp. 890–909). Burlington, MA: Jones & Bartlett Learning.

Vrijens, B., De Geest, S., Hughes, D. A., Przemyslaw, K., Demonceau, J., Ruppar, T., . . . Urquhart, J. (2012). A new taxonomy for describing and defining adherence to medications. *British Journal of Clinical Pharmacology, 73*, 691–705. http://dx.doi.org/10.1111/j.1365-2125.2012.04167.x

Wagena, E. J., Huibers, M. J., & van Schayck, C. P. (2001). Antidepressants in the treatment of patients with COPD: Possible associations between smoking cigarettes, COPD and depression. *Thorax, 56*, 587–588. http://dx.doi.org/10.1136/thorax.56.8.587a

Wang, T. W., Asman, K., Gentzke, A. S., Cullen, K. A., Holder-Hayes, E., Reyes-Guzman, C., . . . King, B. A. (2018). Tobacco product use among adults—United States, 2017. *Morbidity and Mortality Weekly Report, 67*, 1225–1232. http://dx.doi.org/10.15585/mmwr.mm6744a2

Ware, J. E., & Sherbourne, C. D. (1992). The MOS 36-item short-form health survey (SF-36): I. Conceptual framework and item selection. *Medical Care, 30*, 473–483.

Watkins, M. L., Wilcox, T. K., Tabberer, M., Brooks, J. M., Donohue, J. F., Anzueto, A., . . . Crim, C. (2013). Shortness of Breath with Daily Activities Questionnaire: Validation and responder thresholds in patients with chronic obstructive pulmonary disease. *BMJ Open, 3*, e003048. http://dx.doi.org/10.1136/bmjopen-2013-003048

WebMD. (n.d.-a). *Cystic fibrosis*. Retrieved from https://www.webmd.com/children/understanding-cystic-fibrosis-basics

WebMD. (n.d.-b). *Lung diseases overview*. Retrieved from http://www.webmd.com/lung/lung-diseases-overview#1

Weinberger, S. E., Cockrill, B. A., & Mandel, J. (2019). *Principles of pulmonary medicine* (7th ed.). Philadelphia, PA: Elsevier.

Wheaton, A. G., Liu, Y., Croft, J. B., VanFrank, B., Croxton, T. L., Punturieri, A., . . . Greenlund, K. J. (2019). Chronic obstructive pulmonary disease and smoking status—United States, 2017. *Morbidity and Mortality Weekly Report, 68*, 533–538. Retrieved from https://www.cdc.gov/mmwr/volumes/68/wr/mm6824a1.htm

Willgoss, T. G., & Yohannes, A. M. (2013). Anxiety disorders in patients with COPD: A systematic review. *Respiratory Care, 58*, 858–866.

Willgoss, T. G., Yohannes, A. M., Goldbart, J., & Fatoye, F. (2012). "Everything was spiraling out of control": Experiences of anxiety in people with chronic obstructive pulmonary disease. *Heart & Lung, 41*, 562–571. http://dx.doi.org/10.1016/j.hrtlng.2012.07.003

Witkiewitz, K., & Marlatt, G. A. (2007). Overview of relapse prevention. In K. A. Witkiewitz & G. A. Marlatt (Eds.), *Therapist's guide to evidence-based relapse prevention* (pp. 3–17). San Diego, CA: Elsevier Academic Press. Retrieved from http://dx.doi.org/10.1016/B978-012369429-4/50031-8

World Health Organization. (2015). *Human genomics in global health.* Retrieved from https://www.who.int/genomics/public/geneticdiseases/en/index2.html

Yaqoob, Z. J., Al-Kindi, S. G., & Zein, J. G. (2017). Trends and disparities in hospice use among patients dying of COPD in the United States. *Chest, 151,* 1183–1184. http://dx.doi.org/10.1016/j.chest.2017.02.030

Yi, S. W., Hong, J. S., Ohrr, H., & Yi, J. J. (2014). Agent Orange exposure and disease prevalence in Korean Vietnam veterans: The Korean Veterans Health Study. *Environmental Research, 133,* 56–65. http://dx.doi.org/10.1016/j.envres.2014.04.027

Yi, S. W., Ohrr, H., Hong, J. S., & Yi, J. J. (2013). Agent Orange exposure and prevalence of self-reported diseases in Korean Vietnam veterans. *Journal of Preventive Medicine and Public Health, 46,* 213–225. http://dx.doi.org/10.3961/jpmph.2013.46.5.213

Yohannes, A. M., & Alexopoulos, G. S. (2014a). Depression and anxiety in patients with COPD. *European Respiratory Review, 23,* 345–349. http://dx.doi.org/10.1183/09059180.00007813

Yohannes, A. M., & Alexopoulos, G. S. (2014b). Pharmacological treatment of depression in older patients with chronic obstructive pulmonary disease: Impact on the course of the disease and health outcomes. *Drugs & Aging, 31,* 483–492. http://dx.doi.org/10.1007/s40266-014-0186-0

Yohannes, A. M., Kaplan, A., & Hanania, N. A. (2018). COPD in primary care: Key considerations for optimized management: Anxiety and depression in chronic obstructive pulmonary disease: Recognition and management. *The Journal of Family Practice, 67,* S11–S18.

Yohannes, A. M., Willgoss, T. G., Fatoye, F. A., Dip, M. D., & Webb, K. (2012). Relationship between anxiety, depression, and quality of life in adult patients with cystic fibrosis. *Respiratory Care, 57,* 550–556. http://dx.doi.org/10.4187/respcare.01328

Yorke, J., Moosavi, S. H., Shuldham, C., & Jones, P. W. (2010). Quantification of dyspnoea using descriptors: Development and initial testing of the Dyspnoea-12. *Thorax, 65,* 21–26. http://dx.doi.org/10.1136/thx.2009.118521

Zein, J. G., & Erzurum, S. C. (2015). Asthma is different in women. *Current Allergy and Asthma Reports, 15,* 28. http://dx.doi.org/10.1007/s11882-015-0528-y

Index

About the Author

Susan M. Labott, PhD, ABPP, received her doctorate in clinical psychology from Northern Illinois University and completed a postdoctoral fellowship at Henry Ford Hospital. While at the University of Illinois Hospital and Health Sciences System, she developed and directed the Health Psychology Service for 18 years. She is currently professor emerita of clinical psychology in psychiatry. Board certified in clinical health psychology by the American Board of Professional Psychology, she also has interests in ethics and chairs the Social/Behavioral Institutional Review Board at the University of Illinois at Chicago.

About the Series Editor

Ellen A. Dornelas, PhD, is the director for the cancer care delivery and disparities research office at Hartford HealthCare Cancer Institute in Connecticut and associate professor of clinical medicine at the University of Connecticut School of Medicine. Dr. Dornelas received her degree in health psychology from Ferkauf Graduate School of Psychology, Yeshiva University, New York, New York. She has focused her career on the integration of practice and research in clinical health psychology. A practicing psychotherapist, Dr. Dornelas is recognized for her expertise in treating people with heart disease as well as cancer. She has supervised and mentored students for over 2 decades. She has authored multiple books and journal articles and is a featured guest expert on APA's Psychotherapy Video Series. Dr. Dornelas is a Fellow of the American Psychological Association's Division 29 (Society for the Advancement of Psychotherapy).